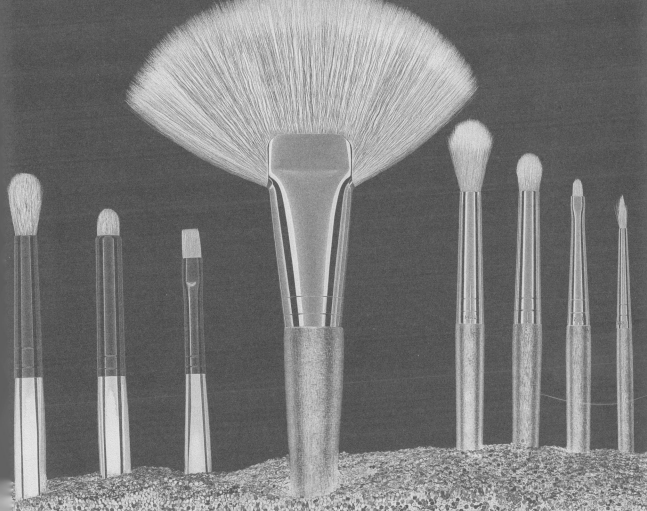

TONI MALT

TRANSFORM

1 MODEL
60 MAKEUP LOOKS

ASSOULINE

Endpages: Toni's must-have brushes,
photo © Adam Browning-Hill.

© 2017 Assouline Publishing
3 Park Avenue, 27th floor
New York, NY 10016, USA
Tel.: 212-989-6769 Fax: 212-647-0005
www.assouline.com
ISBN: 9781614286608

Art direction: Camille Dubois
Designer: Charlotte Sivrière
Editorial direction: Esther Kremer
Editor: Lindsey Tulloch
Color separation by CP Printing
Printed in Italy by Grafiche Milani

TONI MALT

TRANSFORM

1 MODEL
60 MAKEUP LOOKS

ASSOULINE

Table of Contents

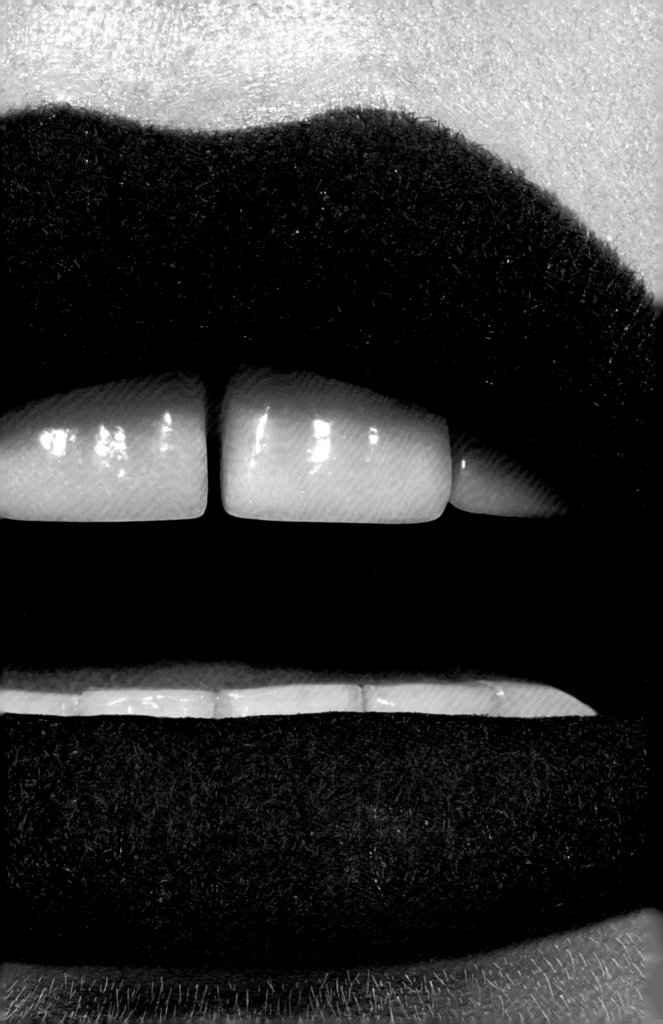

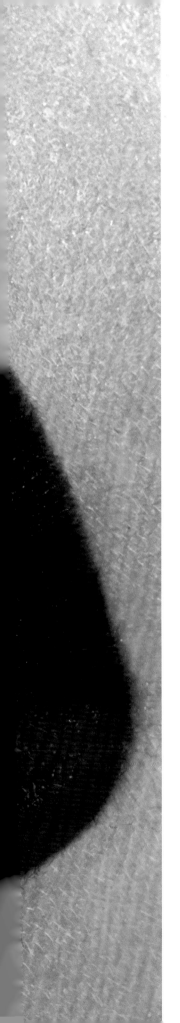

Introduction

Transform is an honest, informative, and mesmerizingly beautiful look into the world of an editorial makeup artist. Combining a love of art with impeccable color skills and vast product knowledge, makeup artist Toni Malt has transformed one model into sixty stunning editorial characters.

A self-confessed team player, Toni firmly believes in passing on her wisdom. "I love working as a team and sharing in success," she says. "I also love sharing knowledge; it's why I wanted to do this book."

Within the pages of *Transform*, Toni shares her well-honed methods, insider insights, and on-the-job tips so aspiring makeup artists can adopt and replicate them.

"What I love most about my job is its power to change," says Toni. "I want to share my skills and demonstrate the tools, products, and techniques that really work."

Meet Sophia

For me, the greatest beauty models are defined as much by their character as by their beauty. A great face structure is key—as are beautiful cheekbones, healthy skin, full lips, and beautiful almond-shaped eyes that take eye makeup well. But it goes so much deeper than that. A great beauty model needs to believe in her expressions, play her character with conviction, and have that special something that keeps you wanting to know more about her.

Sophia is incredibly beautiful, but it's her charm and versatility that draw you in. Shooting the sixty different makeup looks for *Transform* was a lot to ask, but nothing fazed her. She has this incredible ability to morph herself into any character she's asked to become.

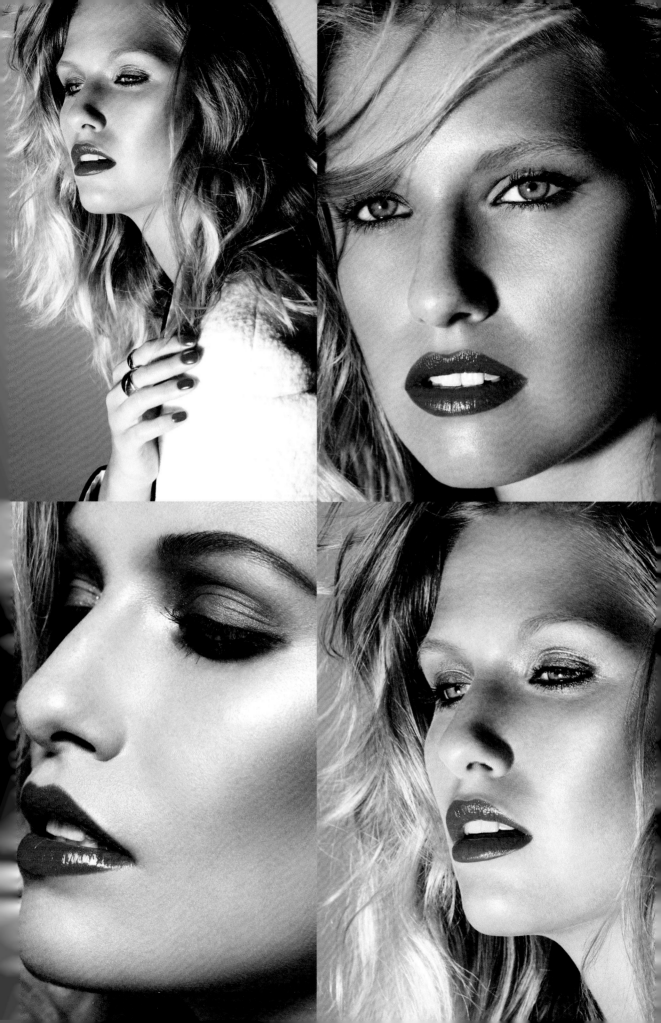

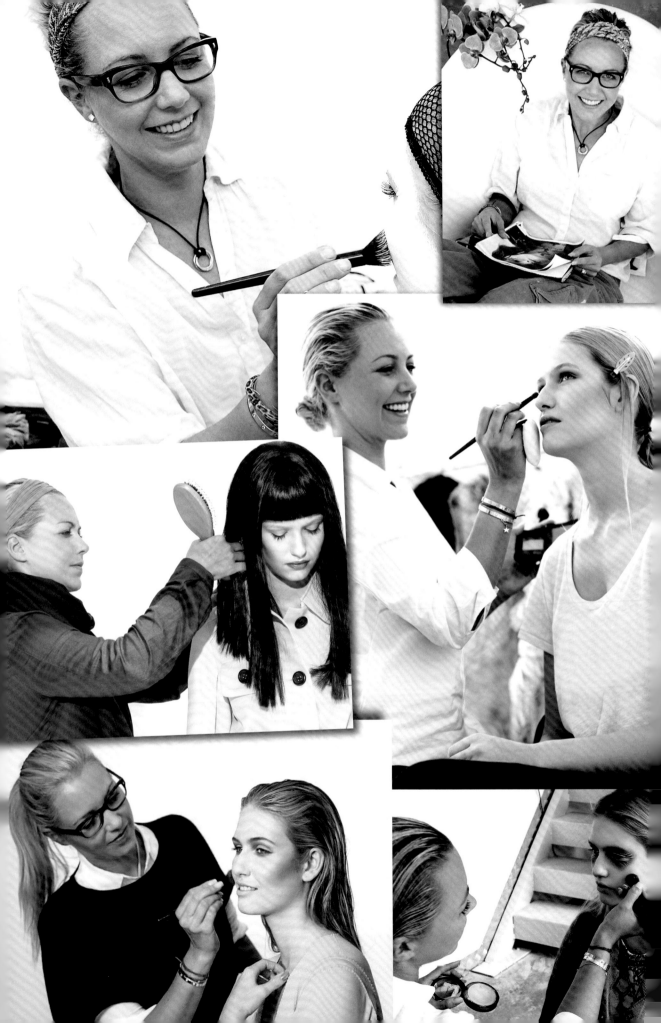

About Toni

Toni Malt is a passionate and gifted makeup artist with an innate talent for creating extraordinarily beautiful faces. From minimalistic looks to freestyle artistic creations, Toni's creative work has been published in top international fashion magazines including *Vogue*, *Elle*, *L'Officiel*, *Marie Claire*, *Harper's Bazaar*, *Grazia*, *Cosmopolitan*, and *Rolling Stone*. She also runs her own makeup academy in Dubai.

Born and raised in Germany, Toni has traveled extensively throughout her career, which spans over a decade. Having lived in both London and New York, she is currently based in Dubai, a city that has proven a great inspiration.

An award-winning makeup artist with covetable contracts with fashion brands, Toni is happiest when in the process of creation, from the initial research right through to shoot day. After years of both organized and on-the-job training, Toni firmly believes in passionately passing on her wisdom. "There is great power in skill and knowledge, and I want to share that with aspiring makeup artists," she says. This desire to share and teach has been a major influence on the creation of *Transform*.

www.tonimalt.com

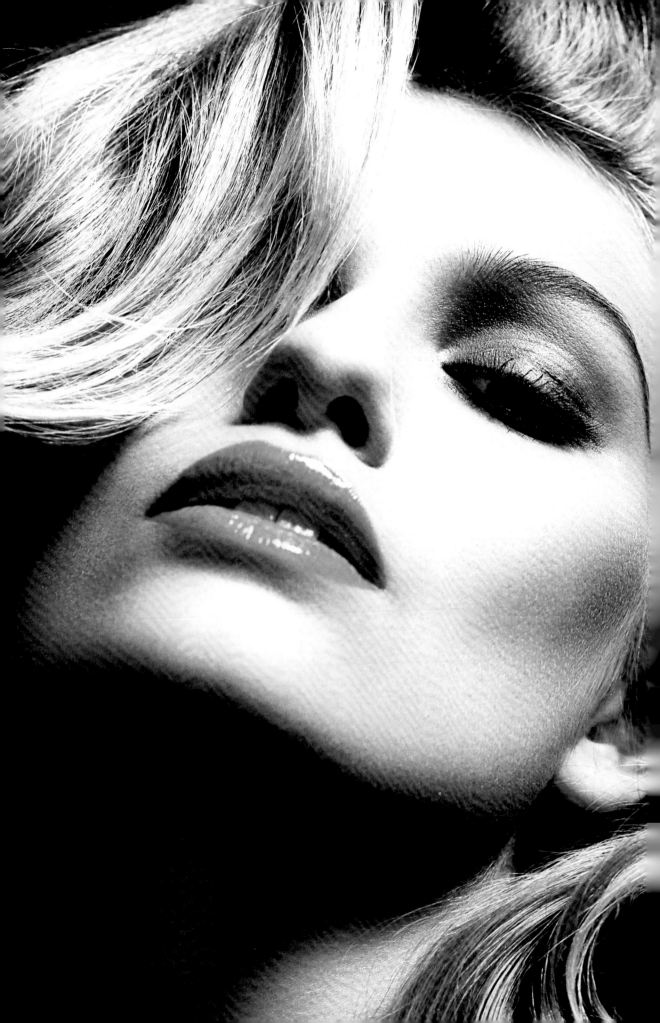

LOOKS

Spellbound

Fairy-tale styling calls for soft, perfectly blended makeup with a touch of magical allure. Eyes take on a whimsical feel with gold highlights and crystal embellishment, while skin stays warm and ethereal with sweeps of pink.

BASE
MAC Pro Full Coverage in NC20. Several layers of Make Up For Ever HD Powder to achieve a velvet finish.

CONTOUR
MAC Powder Blush in Taupe under the cheekbones, then Chanel Joues Contraste in 72 Rose Initial to enhance.

EYES
Blend MAC Matte Eye Shadows in Charcoal Brown and Brun to create a soft smoky eye, followed by one coat of black mascara to enhance the eyelashes (overly strong lashes will diminish the impact of the gold highlight). Illamasqua Liquid Metal in Solstice to highlight the inner corners. Crystals from Make Up For Ever. DUO eyelash adhesive.

EYEBROWS
MAC Eye Brows pencils in Lingering and Fling.

LIPS
MAC Lip Pencil in Subculture to even out the lip line (this is one of my favorite nude lip liners), finished off with plenty of Dior Addict Lip Maximizer, which photographs slightly pink.

To bring this very soft blended makeup to life, the two key elements are the gold highlights and the pink blush. For the gold highlights, I used an amazing product from Illamasqua called Liquid Metal in Solstice.

I applied the gold to the inner corners of the eyes, above the pupil, and halfway below the lower lashes—to create a look that feels organic and real, I placed the gold ever so slightly asymmetrically. I also used the Liquid Metal to set a highlight on the Cupid's bow and in the middle of the chin, which helped unite the eyes with the rest of the face.

To emphasize the abstract idea of this makeup, I used Chanel Joues Contraste (a soft pink blush) in 72 Rose Initial to contour the face around the cheeks, below the chin, and around the jawline. I also applied the blush up into the temples and hairline, to the brow bones, and below the eyes.

I build color slowly and blend well to achieve a soft and ethereal feel. To get the perfect amount of product, I fill my brush with product, then bang the brush handle hard on my makeup table to remove any excess.

As a final touch, I decided to add a tiny crystal below each pupil. Here, I used crystals from Make Up For Ever—the smaller the crystal, the better—and glued them into place using DUO eyelash adhesive.

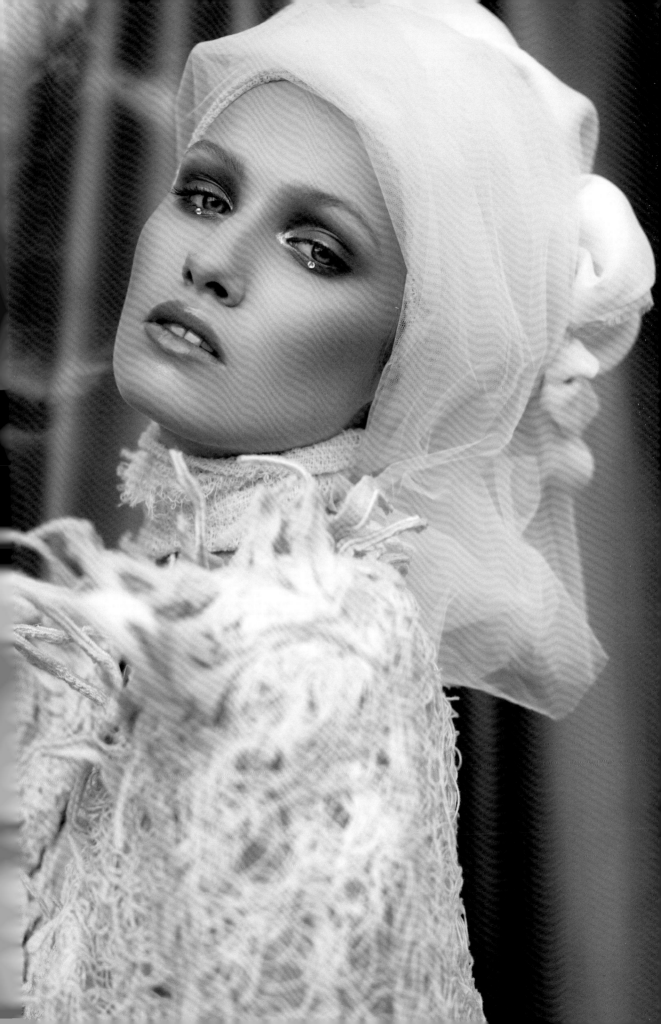

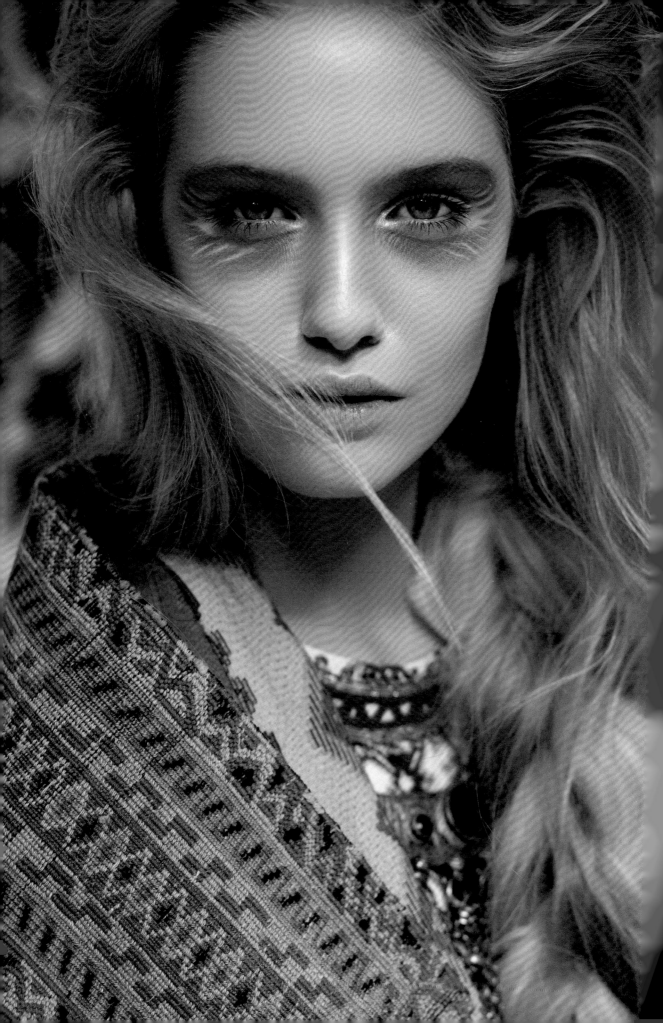

Wild Thing

THERE'S NOTHING DEMURE ABOUT THIS LOOK ORIGINALLY CREATED BY MAKEUP ARTIST EXTRAORDINAIRE RAE MORRIS. BLENDING NEW-AGE AIRBRUSHING TECHNIQUES WITH TRADITIONAL MAKEUP METHODS, THIS IS FIERCENESS AT ITS MOST FLAWLESS.

BASE
Charlotte Tilbury Light Wonder in Fair 2.
Charlotte Tilbury Airbrush Flawless Finish in 1 Fair to set.

CONTOUR
Illamasqua Powder Blush in Disobey.

EYES
MAC Pro Paint Stick in Primary Yellow.
Temptu Air Compressor with SP-35 Airbrush and S/B Adjuster in Red.
Becca Shimmering Skin Perfector Pressed Highlighter in Pearl on the inner corners of the eyes.
MAC Eye Kohl in Fascinating. Black mascara on the top and bottom lashes.

LIPS
I applied whatever foundation was left on the brush over the lips. After a few minutes this dried-out effect appeared, which I thought worked really well.

THIS AIRBRUSHED TECHNIQUE WAS FIRST PIONEERED BY THE AMAZING MAKEUP ARTIST RAE MORRIS, MAKEUP DIRECTOR AT L'ORÉAL PARIS AND AUTHOR OF MAKEUP BOOKS SUCH AS QUICK LOOKS AND EXPRESS MAKEUP. I HAVE ALWAYS LOVED RAE'S WORK; IT'S CRISP, MODERN, AND SEXY WITH FLAWLESS FINISHING, AND HER ENDLESS DESIRE TO EXPERIMENT WITH METHODS IS INSPIRING. TO SEE HOW RAE DOES THIS TECHNIQUE, WATCH HER YOUTUBE VIDEO TUTORIAL ON HER "MOTHMAN" LOOK—IT'S HOW I INITIALLY DISCOVERED THE TECHNIQUE.

USING A SEPHORA PRO AIRBRUSH CONCEALER BRUSH 57, I APPLIED THE BASE COLOR (MAC PRO PAINT STICK IN PRIMARY YELLOW), BLENDING SOFTLY OUTWARD ON AND AROUND THE EYES. I THEN ASKED SOPHIA TO SCRUNCH UP HER EYES AS TIGHTLY AS POSSIBLE. WHILE SHE DID THIS, I USED MY TEMPTU AIR COMPRESSOR AIRBRUSH TO PAINT S/B ADJUSTER IN RED OVER THE SAME AREA, SOFTLY BLENDING OUTWARD. THE MOMENT SOPHIA OPENED HER EYES, THESE UNIQUE PATTERNS APPEARED ON HER FACE. THEY LOOK ALMOST LIKE FEATHER STROKES—JUST SO PRETTY! TO ADD DEFINITION TO THE EYES, I APPLIED MAC EYE KOHL IN FASCINATING AND A SINGLE COAT OF BLACK MASCARA TO BOTH THE TOP AND BOTTOM LASHES. I THEN FINISHED WITH BECCA SHIMMERING SKIN PERFECTOR PRESSED HIGHLIGHTER IN PEARL TO HIGHLIGHT THE INNER CORNERS OF THE EYES.

BE AWARE THAT THIS LOOK DOES NOT WORK ON EVERY MODEL; SOME MODELS CREATE THE PERFECT WRINKLES AND SOME DON'T. THIS IS DIFFICULT TO PREDICT, SO I SUGGEST DOING A TRIAL WITH YOUR MODEL BEFORE THE SHOOT OR HAVING A PLAN B READY IN CASE IT DOESN'T LOOK GREAT—A BACKUP PLAN IS ALWAYS WISE WHEN DOING MORE ADVANCED TECHNIQUES. I USED THIS SAME TECHNIQUE A COUPLE WEEKS LATER FOR A DRUGSTORE CAMPAIGN AND IT JUST DIDN'T WORK, SO I ENDED UP DOING AN AIRBRUSHED GRADATION OF PINKS AND YELLOWS ACROSS THE EYES, INTO THE TEMPLES, AND DOWN THE CHEEKS. IT LOOKED JUST AS BEAUTIFUL.

High Drama

Seduction goes into overdrive as the 1940s screen siren gets a modern update. Porcelain skin, subtle contouring, and a high-shine pout get top billing.

BASE
Charlotte Tilbury Light Wonder Foundation in Fair 2. Make Up For Ever HD Powder across the T-zone.

HIGHLIGHT
Skin N Nature Cookie Marble Blusher in 01 Rose.

EYES
Elizabeth Arden Eight Hour Cream. Bobbi Brown Eye Shadow in Tan in the creases. Becca Shimmering Skin Perfector Pressed Highlighter in Pearl to highlight the inner corners. MAC 30 Lash single lashes in Medium and Long. Black mascara.

CONTOUR
Bobbi Brown Eye Shadow in Tan.

EYEBROWS
MAC Eye Brows pencils in Lingering and Stud.

LIPS
MAC Lip Pencil in Beet, MAC Lipstick in Hang Up, and MAC Clear Lipglass.

I loved doing this makeup; it's so clean yet so expressive and oh so elegant. This early 1940s film noir makeup interpretation is best achieved by keeping the skin clean with the smallest amount of contour. I created the contour using Bobbi Brown Eye Shadow in Tan—the same product that I used on the eyes.

To achieve these sophisticated eyes, I added a small dab of Elizabeth Arden Eight Hour Cream to the eyelids, on top of the Bobbi Brown Eye Shadow in Tan in the creases. I enhanced the inner corners of the eyes with Becca Shimmering Skin Perfector Pressed Highlighter in Pearl, then finished them off by adding lots of MAC 30 Lash single lashes in Medium to the top curve of the eye and in Long at the outer corners to elongate the eyes. I then applied one coat of black mascara. To emphasize the eyes and frame the face, I darkened the eyebrows slightly and elongated them.

To give this look that true early-1940s film noir feeling, I chose a stunning blue-red lipstick by MAC called Hang Up, then added a coat of MAC Clear Lipglass to the bottom lip to give the lips an edgy elegance boost.

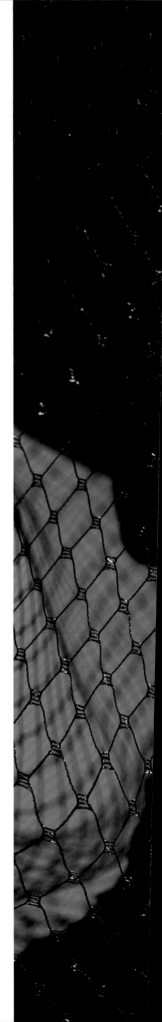

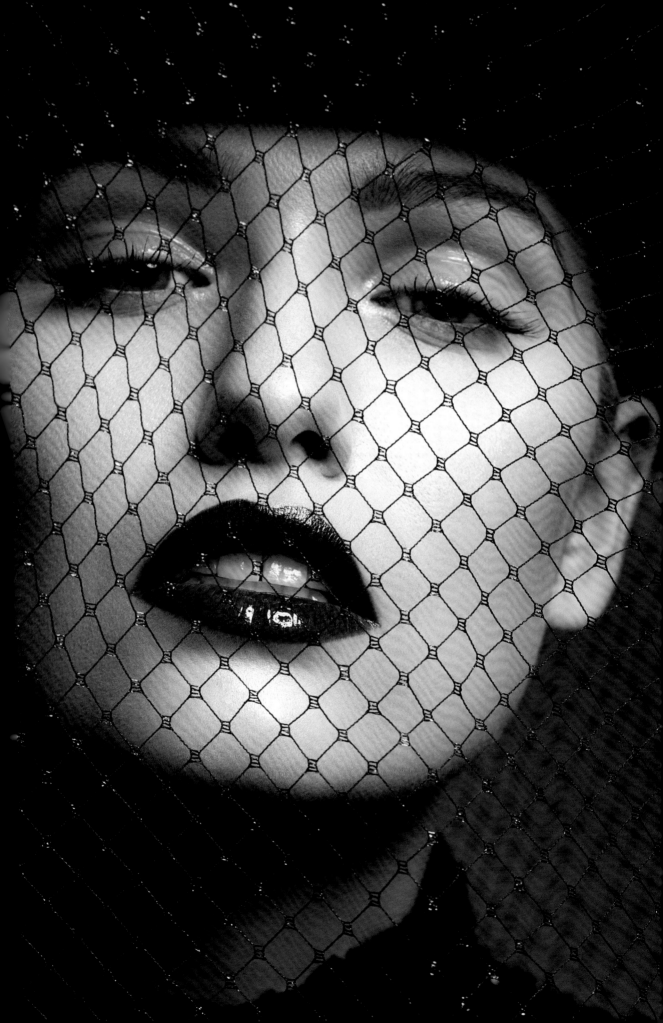

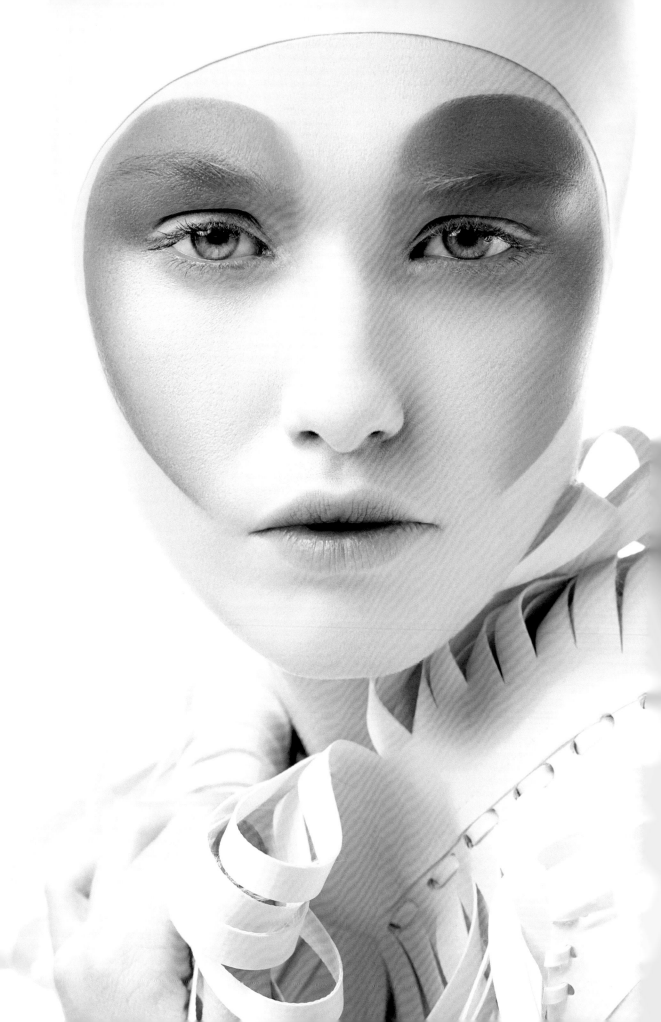

Ultra Violet

Designer Michael Cinco's stunning avant-garde style calls for makeup that's truly otherworldly. For this mythical transformation, stencils and standout color are key.

BASE
MAC Pro Full Coverage Foundation in W10 blended with MAC Pro Full Coverage Foundation in White.
Make Up For Ever HD Powder to set.

FACE PAINT
MAC Pro Paint Sticks in Hi-Def Cyan and French Violet.

EYES
MAC Pro Paint Sticks in Hi-Def Cyan and French Violet applied down to the creases.
Eyelids are left color free with only the foundation base.

LIPS
MAC Pro Paint Stick in French Violet dabbed in with the finger.

STENCILS
Cut out from a blank sheet of paper. Surgical tape.

I love painting and the transformation it can achieve—holding a brush in my hand makes me so happy! MAC Paint Sticks are one of my favorite products. They were perfect for this look because they're highly pigmented and so easy to blend; the finished effect is like real skin.

I kept my foundation really light in color to create a high contrast and allow the soft cyan and violet to really pop. To make the stencil, I cut a half-moon shape out of a blank sheet of A4 paper, making slight adjustments along the way by placing it against Sophia's face. Once I had the shape, I attached the stencil to one side of Sophia's head with surgical tape.

I started adding color by using a MAC 217 brush to apply MAC Pro Paint Stick in Hi-Def Cyan underneath the eyes. Then, using an Illamasqua Blusher Brush (my favorite brush when using MAC Paint Sticks), I blended color onto the cheeks starting from below the pupils out toward the side of the face into the stencil. I then worked the French Violet Paint Stick into the skin, stippling it from the stencil corners slowly inward until I had a blended graduation of color. To set and mattify the makeup, I dusted the color with Make Up For Ever HD Powder.

The key to this look is symmetry. To achieve this, only make a stencil for half of the face. It can then be flipped to create the other side—this will guarantee that both sides are identical.

Starlight

STAR LIGHT, STAR BRIGHT... SEND YOUR LOOK DIRECTLY
INTO THE GALAXY WITH A STAR DUSTING OF FULL BODY GLITTER
IT'S ALL ABOUT SPARKLE AND DAZZLING SHINE.

SKIN
Kryolan Glitter Gel in Clear.

GLITTER
One pot of MAC 3D Glitter
in Silver.
Half a pot of Make Up For
Ever Extra Large Size
Glitter in White.
Half a large tube of arts-and-
crafts glitter in silver.
MAC 187 Duo Fibre Face Brush.

TO ADD DEPTH AND VARIETY IN THE REFLECTION, I STARTED THIS LOOK BY MIXING THREE DIFFERENT TYPES OF GLITTER ON A PLATE. I THEN PREPPED THE SKIN BY APPLYING KRYOLAN GLITTER GEL IN CLEAR SECTION BY SECTION—STARTING WITH THE FACE, FOLLOWED BY THE NECK AND SHOULDERS—WITH A LARGE, FLAT FOUNDATION BRUSH. THERE ARE MANY PRODUCTS YOU CAN USE TO ADHERE GLITTER TO THE FACE, BUT I PREFER KRYOLAN GLITTER GEL BECAUSE IT'S REALLY GENTLE ON THE SKIN AND THE GLITTER ADHERES TO IT PERFECTLY.

TO APPLY THE GLITTER, I USED A MAC 187 DUO FIBRE FACE BRUSH, WHICH I DIPPED INTO THE PLATE OF MIXED GLITTER BEFORE GENTLY PRESSING ONTO THE GLUE-PREPPED SKIN. THE KEY IS TO NOT PRESS THE BRUSH MORE THAN TWICE OVER THE SAME AREA, AS THIS WILL MATTIFY THE GLITTER AND DIMINISH ITS REFLECTION. ONCE THE GLITTER COVERED THE MODEL'S EXPOSED SKIN, I ADDED SHAPE TO THE FACE BY ADDING MAC 3D GLITTER IN SILVER TO THE PARTS OF THE SKIN THAT I WOULD NORMALLY HIGHLIGHT—AREAS SUCH AS THE INNER CORNERS OF THE EYES, THE CUPID'S BOW, THE MIDDLE OF THE CHIN, THE CHEEKBONES, AND THE EYELIDS.

BE AWARE THAT ABOUT HALF OF THE GLITTER SEEMS TO DISAPPEAR THE MOMENT IT'S PHOTOGRAPHED, SO MAKE SURE YOU HAVE CREATED A VERY EVEN GLITTER COVERAGE, USING DOUBLE THE AMOUNT YOU THINK YOU NEED.

WITH GLITTER LOOKS SUCH AS THIS ONE, IT'S IMPORTANT TO TAKE GREAT CARE OF YOUR MODEL'S SKIN. THE GLITTER TENDS TO PINCH THE SKIN AFTER ABOUT TEN MINUTES AND WILL OFTEN CAUSE A MODEL'S SKIN TO BECOME ITCHY AND UNCOMFORTABLE. MAKE SURE YOU ARE WELL EQUIPPED TO CLEANSE YOUR MODEL'S SKIN BY HAVING A LARGE TOWEL, GENTLE SOAP, AND A GOOD-QUALITY CLEANSING PRODUCT ON HAND. ALSO HAVE SURGICAL TAPE ACCESSIBLE TO REMOVE ANY LITTLE PATCHES OF LEFTOVER GLITTER—SIMPLY STICK THE TAPE OVER THE GLITTER SPOT, THEN SLOWLY PEEL AWAY. REMEMBER TO REHYDRATE YOUR MODEL'S SKIN POST-SHOOT WITH A TEN-MINUTE MASK FOLLOWED BY MOISTURIZER.

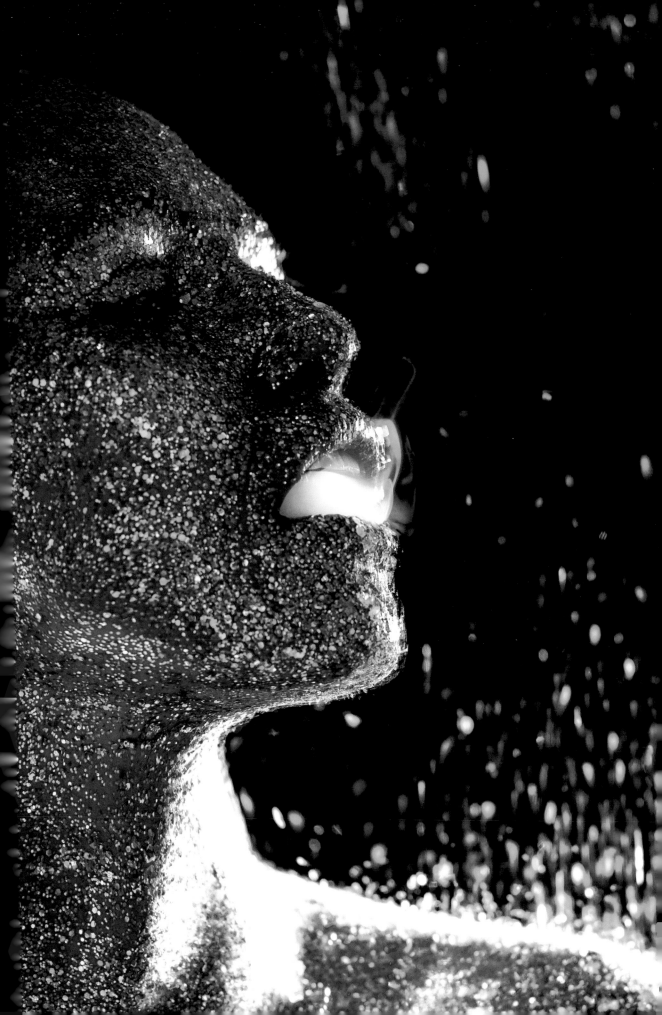

"Make it your goal to apply the least amount of product to achieve the greatest effect. It's the most important key in achieving modern makeup."

Toni Malt

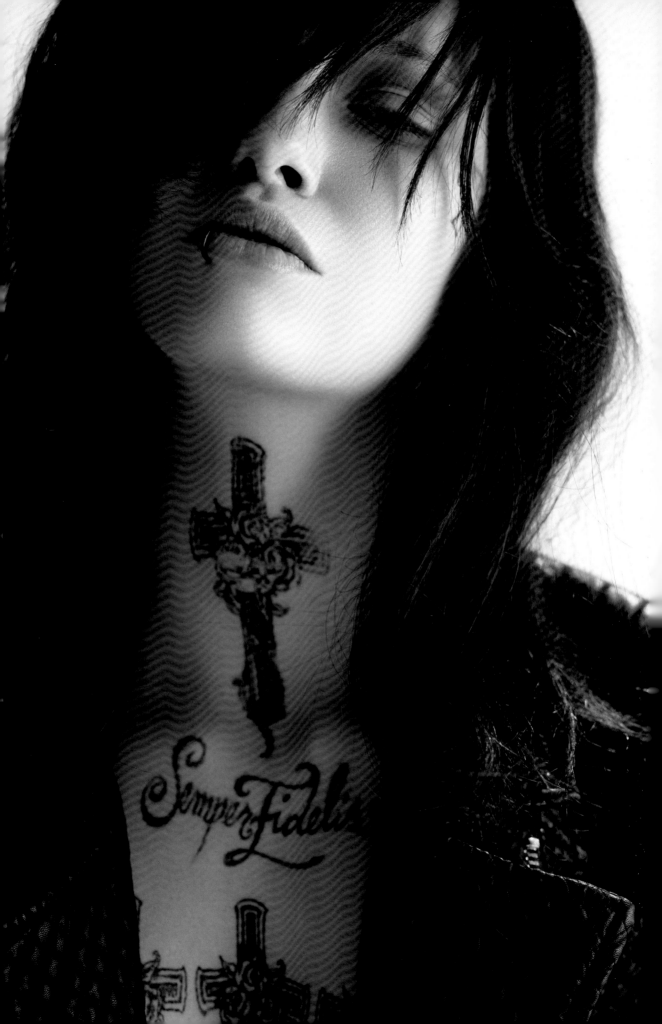

Rebel Ink

TAKE A WALK ON THE DARK SIDE WITH ATTITUDE-HEAVY TEMPORARY TRANSFER TATTOOS. THIS IS BEAUTY AT ITS MOST HARDCORE.

BASE
Very little MAC Pro Full Coverage in NC20 applied with a moist Beauty Blender.

EYES
MAC Matte Eye Shadow in Cork in the creases and below the eyes.
Becca Shimmering Skin Perfector Pressed Highlighter in Pearl to brighten the inner corners of the eyes.
Eyelashes were left natural with no mascara.

LIPS
Elizabeth Arden Eight Hour Cream.
Becca Shimmering Skin Perfector Pressed Highlighter in Pearl on the Cupid's bow.

TATTOOS
Temptu Pro Transfer Tattoos.
Johnson & Johnson Baby Oil.
70% isopropyl alcohol.
Cotton balls.
Make Up For Ever HD Powder.

FOR THIS LOOK, I USED FIVE FLOWERED CROSSES, A SCRIPT TATTOO (SEMPER FIDELIS MEANS "ALWAYS FAITHFUL"), AND A TINY CROSS, WHICH I USED ON THE FACE. APPLYING TRANSFER TATTOOS CAN TAKE A BIT OF PRACTICE, SO I RECOMMEND HAVING A FEW SPARES SO YOU CAN PERFECT YOUR TECHNIQUE ON YOUR OWN SKIN BEFORE WORKING ON A MODEL. I RIPPED THE FIRST CROSS I APPLIED ON MYSELF, BUT THE SECOND ONE WENT ON PERFECTLY.

IN ORDER TO PLACE MULTIPLE TATTOOS NEXT TO EACH OTHER, I NEEDED TO SEE EXACTLY WHERE ONE TATTOO ENDED AND THE NEXT ONE BEGAN. TO DO THIS, I CUT OUT EACH OF THE TATTOOS APPROXIMATELY ONE CENTIMETER AWAY FROM THE DESIGN. BEFORE APPLYING THE TATTOOS, I CLEANED THE AREAS OF SKIN WHERE I WANTED TO STICK THE TRANSFERS WITH A COTTON BALL SOAKED IN 70% ISOPROPYL RUBBING ALCOHOL (YOU CAN BUY THIS AT PHARMACIES). WHILE THE SKIN WAS STILL MOIST, I PLACED THE TRANSFER FACEDOWN IN THE DESIRED POSITION. IT'S IMPORTANT TO PRESS FIRMLY ON THE TRANSFER WITH AN ALCOHOL-SATURATED COTTON BALL UNTIL THE DESIGN SHOWS THROUGH THE BACKING PAPER. ONCE THIS HAPPENED, I PATTED THE TRANSFER WITH MY FINGERS BEFORE PRESSING FIRMLY WITH THE COTTON BALL AGAIN. THE KEY IS TO TAKE YOUR TIME; EACH TATTOO WILL TAKE A MINIMUM OF THREE TO FIVE MINUTES TO TRANSFER.

WHEN YOU THINK THE TRANSFER IS READY, LIFT OFF ONE CORNER OF THE BACKING PAPER WHILE IT'S STILL WET. IF IT HASN'T TRANSFERRED YET, REPEAT THE PROCESS WITH THE COTTON BALL AND ALCOHOL.

ONCE THE TRANSFERRED TATTOOS WERE COMPLETELY DRY (THIS TAKES ABOUT THIRTY SECONDS), I GENTLY PATTED OVER THEM WITH A POWDER PUFF DUSTED WITH A LITTLE MAKE UP FOR EVER HD POWDER. THIS REMOVES ANY SHINE AND MAKES THE TATTOO LOOK MUCH MORE REALISTIC.

TO REMOVE THE TRANSFERS, SIMPLY USE A COTTON BALL SATURATED WITH BABY OIL AND GENTLY WIPE. THE TATTOOS WILL SLIP EASILY OFF THE SKIN.

Ice Queen

Embellished with Swarovski crystals and pearls, these two magical looks take their cues from the wonderful bejeweled creations of Amato Haute Couture. Skin is porcelain perfect so the brows can take center stage.

BASE
MAC Pro Full Coverage in NC20.
Make Up For Ever HD Powder to set the T-zone.

CONTOUR
MAC Powder Blush in Taupe.

HIGHLIGHT
Chanel Poudre Signée de Chanel Illuminating Powder.

EYES
MAC Matte Eye Shadow in Brun to contour the eyes at the creases.
Becca Shimmering Skin Perfetor Pressed Highlighter in Pearl to highlight the eyelids and the inner corners of the eyes.
MAC Matte Eye Shadow in Brun as contour underneath the eyes.
MAC White Eye Kohl in Fascinating applied on the waterlines.
MAC 33 Lash false lashes applied to the top lashes.

A single coat of black mascara.

LIPS
MAC Lip Erase in Pale all over the lips.
Becca Shimmering Skin Perfector Pressed Highlighter in Pearl on the Cupid's bow.

EYEBROWS
Elmer's All Purpose School Glue Stick.
Swarovski crystals.
Swarovski pearls.
DUO eyelash adhesive.

I loved creating these looks. Amato Couture designs are so out-of-this-world beautiful that it's a great challenge to create makeup that does them justice. Amato gave us one dress embellished with crystals and one with pearls for this shoot, so I followed his lead and created crystal eyebrows for the first look and pearl for the second.

To prep the eyebrows, I brushed them with a strong disposable mascara wand in the direction of growth. I then applied two coats of Elmer's All Purpose School Glue Stick. It's important to press hard while applying the glue to ensure all the brow hairs lie flat on the skin and to make sure the first coat has dried completely before applying the second. If your model has very fine eyebrows, this step may not be required.

To apply the crystals, I used DUO eyelash adhesive on top of the glued-down eyebrows. I like to use a variety of crystal sizes; because each crystal reflects the light differently, it gives this look a much more three-dimensional feel.

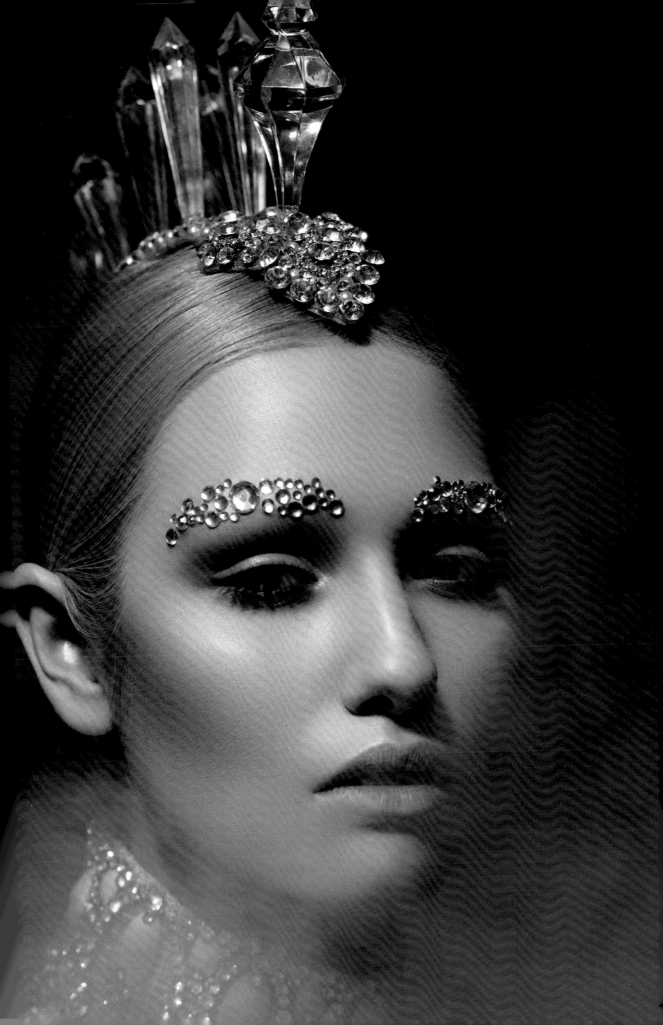

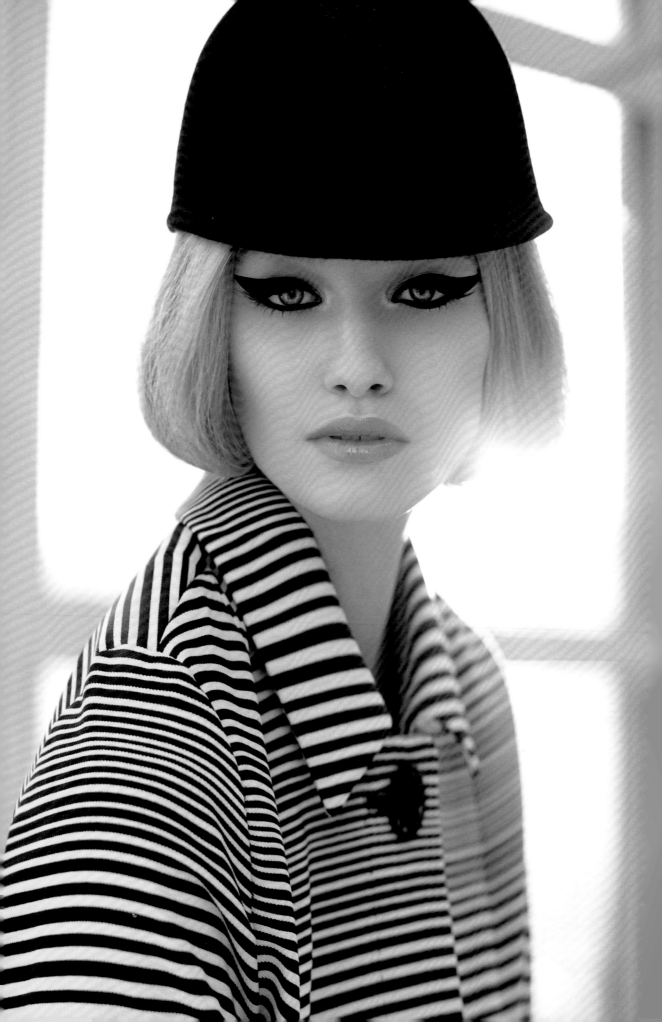

Feline Sleek

A BOLD AND SHARPLY DEFINED CAT EYE IS A TIMELESS WAY TO RAMP UP THE SEX APPEAL.

BASE
MAC Pro Full Coverage in NC20. A little Make Up For Ever HD Powder to set.

HIGHLIGHT
Skin N Nature Cookie Marble Blusher in 01 Rose.

CONTOUR
MAC Sculpting Powder Pro Palettes in Sculpt and Shadowy.

EYES
Chanel Écriture de Chanel Eyeliner Pen in 10 Noir. Yaby es053 Rose Wood Eye Shadow (from the Yaby Dramatically Neutral palette) in the creases and below the lower lashes. MAC Eye Kohl in Smolder. MAC 45 Lash and lots of black mascara.

EYEBROWS
Using a mascara wand, brush a small amount of MAC Pro Full Coverage in NC15 through the eyebrows to lighten them (too much product will clump the brow hairs).

LIPS
MAC Lip Pencil in Naked. Rimmel Lasting Finish Matte Lipstick by Kate Moss in 25. MAC Clear Lipglass to enhance.

I love a crisp, exaggerated feline eye; it's so bold, gutsy, and sexy while still looking really serene and innocent. The size of the cat-eye shape will depend on the eye shape of your model; I needed to go this big on Sophia's eyes to ensure I had a clean, smooth line. Hooded eyes tend to need this size of wing, but it's possible to create a smaller shape for other eye shapes—the rule is that you need to be able to see the eyeliner on top of the moving eyelid.

After finishing my foundation, I used Chanel's Écriture de Chanel in Noir to map out my shape—remember to ask your model to close her eyes until the eyeliner has dried! I like to do the eyeliner before I do any other eye makeup—that way, I can correct mistakes without destroying anything beneath. Once I had created the shape, I cleaned up the lines and filled it all in. I can't stress enough the importance of taking your time; there is nothing worse than crooked eyeliner. Any mistakes can be cleaned up easily by dipping a pointy cotton swab into thick moisturizer and running it over the error.

Once the eyeliner was dry, I contoured the eye in the creases and below the lower lashes ever so slightly using Yaby es053 Rose Wood Eye Shadow. I then applied a second coat of eyeliner to remove any shadow falloff. To finish, I tightlined (filled in) the top and bottom waterlines with MAC Eye Kohl in Smolder and added a pair of MAC 45 Lashes to emphasize the outer corners of the eyes.

Rockabilly Glamour

Clumpy, spidery, all-out lashes are the focus of this 1960s-inspired rock look. Just as soon as you think you've loaded on enough lashes and mascara, crack open another packet and do another coat. Or three.

BASE
Charlotte Tilbury Light Wonder Foundation in 2 Fair. Make Up For Ever HD Powder.

LIPS
MAC Lip Pencil in Cyber and Illamasqua lipstick in Disciple.

CONTOUR
Dolce & Gabbana The Bronzer in Desert 20.

EYEBROWS
Simply brushed through with a clean mascara wand to keep the focus on the eyes.

EYES
Dolce & Gabbana The Bronzer in Desert 20 to contour the eyes lightly in the creases and below the lower eyelashes. MAC Fluidline in Blacktrack on the top lashes.

Ardell Demi Wispy Lashes in Black.
MAC 30 Lash single lashes in Short, Medium, and Long.
DiorShow Maximizer Lash Plumping Serum.
Black mascara.

The key element to this look is heaps of false eyelashes. More is definitely more here. To create the top lashes, I applied a set of Demi Wispy black strip lashes by Ardell before adding a whole packet of MAC 30 Lash single lashes in Long and Medium over the top. To the bottom lashes, I glued one and a half packets of MAC 30 Lash single lashes in Short, keeping as close as possible to the natural lash lines to make the lashes look realistic.

I then coated the lashes with DiorShow Maximizer Lash Plumping Serum—a white gel that coats the lashes to make them appear incredibly full—followed by layers and layers of black mascara. When I thought I was finished, I asked Sophia to add three more coats of mascara; I had been working on her eyes so long, I felt she needed a break! I love this eye makeup look because the thick lashes throw their own shadow and enhance the contouring already done with eye shadow.

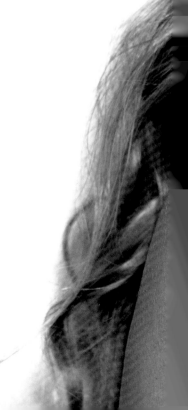

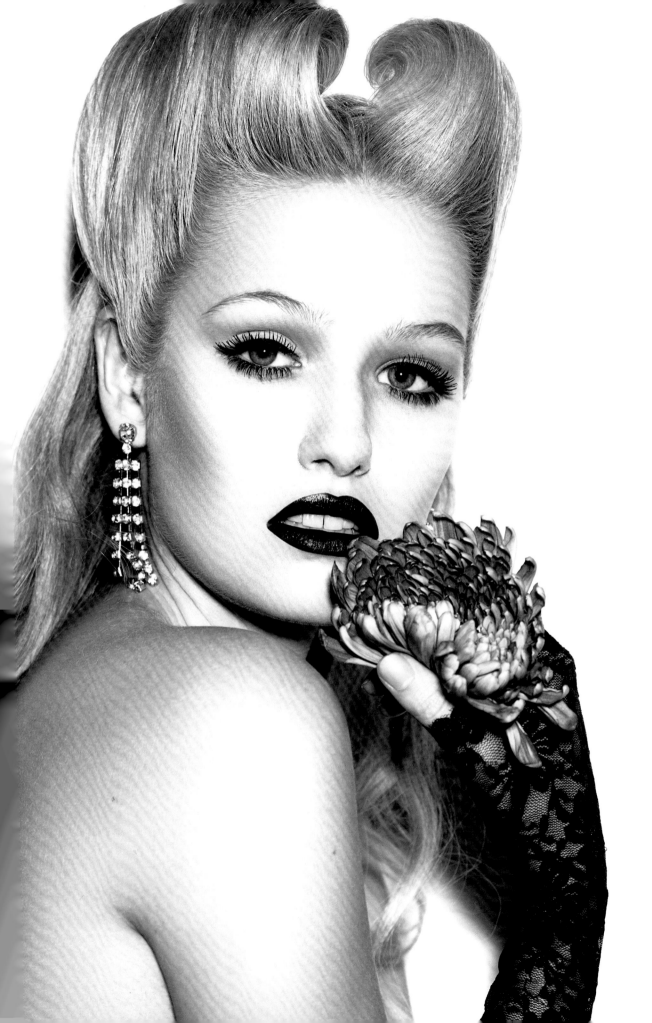

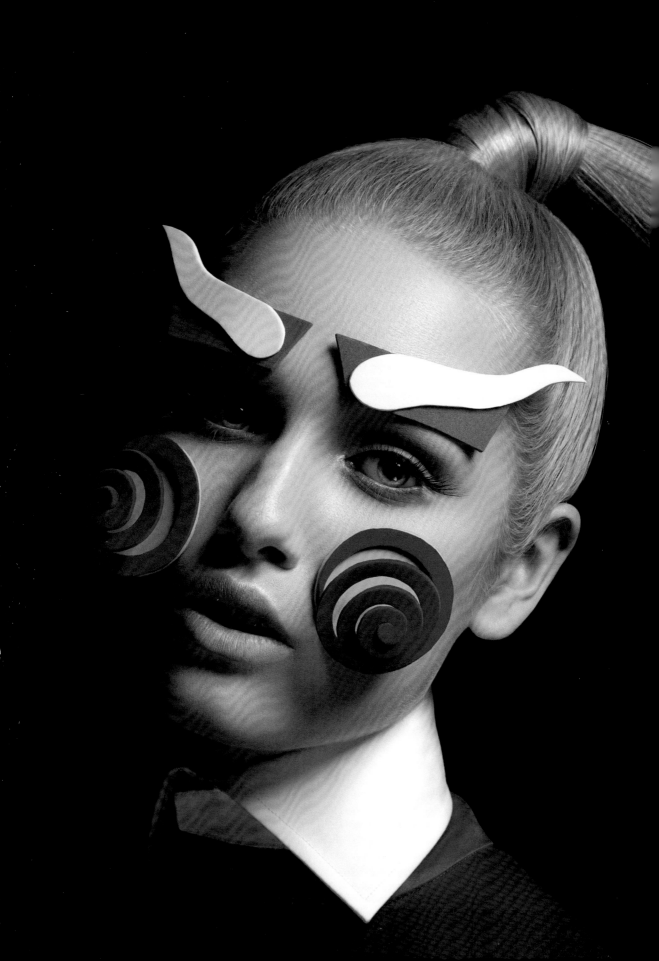

MAKEUP GOES 3-D WITH POP ART-INSPIRED COLORED FOAM CUTOUTS.
THIS LOOK TAKES DIRECTION FROM THE TECHNIQUE ORIGINALLY INVENTED
BY MAKEUP ARTIST LISA ELDRIDGE FOR DANSK MAGAZINE.

BASE
Charlotte Tilbury Light Wonder
Foundation in 4 Fair.
Make Up For Ever HD Powder
to set.

CONTOUR
MAC Powder Blush in Taupe.

LIPS
MAC Lip Erase in Pale dabbed
onto the lips.
Becca Shimmering Skin Perfector
Press Highlighter in Pearl to
highlight the Cupid's bow.

EYES
MAC Powder Blush in Taupe
to contour the creases and
below the lower lashes.
MAC Eye Kohl in Fascinating
to whiten the waterlines.
Girls Aloud Lashes by Eylure
in Nicola on the top lashes
to enhance the eye shape.
Becca Shimmering Skin
Perfector Press Highlighter
in Pearl to highlight the inner

I HAVE ALWAYS LOOKED UP TO LISA ELDRIDGE. AS A MAKEUP ARTIST, SHE IS SUCH AN INCREDIBLE TALENT—HER CREATIVITY AND DEPTH OF KNOWLEDGE MAKE HER ONE OF THE LEADING ARTISTS OF OUR TIME. THE FIRST TIME I SAW CUTOUTS BEING USED IN THIS WAY WAS ON AN EDITORIAL SHOOT SHE DID FOR THE DANISH MAGAZINE DANSK, WHERE SHE USED PAPER CUTOUTS. SHE THEN REIMAGINED THE LOOK LATER IN A CAMPAIGN FOR HARVEY NICHOLS. FOR ALL OF LISA'S TIPS AND TRICKS, CHECK OUT HER BLOG AT WWW.LISAELDRIDGE.COM.

FOR THIS LOOK, I WENT TO AN ARTS AND CRAFTS STORE AND PURCHASED THIN FOAM SHEETS. I OUTLINED THE SHAPES I NEEDED AND MY TEAM AND I CUT THEM OUT DURING OUR LUNCH BREAK ON ONE OF THE SHOOT DAYS. I THEN STACKED AND GLUED THE PIECES OF FOAM TOGETHER USING DUO EYELASH ADHESIVE AND ADHERED THEM TO THE FACE WITH THE GLUE. IT IS SO EASY AND FUN YET SO EFFECTIVE.

Fade to White

SKIN TURNS PORCELAIN PALE WITH CAREFUL LAYERING
OF MOISTURIZER, FOUNDATION, AND JUST A TOUCH OF SHEEN.
A DEFINING MOMENT. THIS ALABASTER-INSPIRED SHOOT
MARKS THE POINT WHEN A MAKEUP ARTIST MEETS HER MUSE.

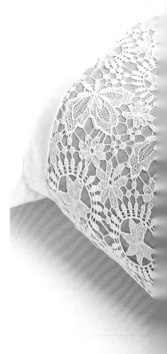

BASE
MAC Pro Full Coverage in
W10. A little Make Up For Ever
HD Powder to set.
Becca Shimmering Skin
Perfector Pressed Highlighter
in Pearl applied sparingly
to add a slight glow.

CONTOUR
MAC Pro Sculpting Cream
in Naturally Defined.
Illamasqua Powder Blusher
in Disobey to set.
A tiny bit of Yaby pp061
Copper Ruby Eye Shadow
(from the Yaby World of Pearl
Paint palette).

EYES
Yaby pp061 Copper Ruby
Eye Shadow (from the Yaby
World of Pearl Paint palette)
to contour the creases and
below the lower eyelashes,
winging both outward toward
the temple.
Yaby pp048 Chocolate
Smoothie (from the Yaby
World of Pearl Paint palette)
to add definition in the creases.
Becca Shimmering Skin
Perfector Pressed Highlighter
in Pearl on the eyelids and
inner corners of the eyes.
MAC Eye Kohl in Fascinating
on the waterlines.

One coat of black mascara
on the top lashes only.

EYEBROWS
MAC Pro Full Coverage
in W10 brushed through
the brows with a mascara
wand to lighten. Keep the
foundation light, as too much
will clump the eyebrow hairs.

LIPS
Becca Shimmering Skin
Perfector Pressed Highlighter
in Pearl on the Cupid's bow,
followed by MAC Pro Lip
Erase in Dim dabbed onto
the lips with a finger.

THIS WAS MY FIRST SHOOT WITH MY MODEL SOPHIA. SHE HAD JUST ARRIVED
IN DUBAI FOR A THREE-MONTH MODEL STAY. I HAD BEEN WAITING FOR
OVER TWO YEARS FOR THE RIGHT MOMENT TO START THIS BOOK AND, AFTER
WORKING WITH SOPHIA ON THIS SHOOT, I KNEW THE MOMENT HAD COME.
I WAS DETERMINED THAT SHE WOULD BE MY MODEL FOR THE "ONE MODEL/
SIXTY LOOKS" CONCEPT. SHE WAS JUST PERFECT!

THE KEY ELEMENT FOR THIS LOOK IS THE ALABASTER-PALE SKIN WITH ITS
BEAUTIFUL SHEEN. IT TAKES TIME TO CREATE AS MOISTURIZER, FOUNDATION, AND
SHEEN NEED TO BE APPLIED TO ALL EXPOSED BODY PARTS. AFTER MOISTURIZING,
I APPLIED MAC PRO FULL COVERAGE IN W10 AS A FOUNDATION TO SOPHIA'S
FACE, NECK, DÉCOLLETAGE, ARMS, AND LEGS. I THEN USED A KABUKI BRUSH
TO APPLY BECCA SHIMMERING SKIN PERFECTOR PRESSED HIGHLIGHTER IN
PEARL ALL OVER THE FOUNDATION TO ACHIEVE AN ETHEREAL SHEEN.

TO GET A LIGHT AND EVEN LUSTER, TAP OFF ANY EXCESS PIGMENT FROM
THE KABUKI BRUSH PRIOR TO EACH APPLICATION. THE LEGS, ARMS, AND
DÉCOLLETAGE ARE JUST AS IMPORTANT AS THE FACE IN THIS LOOK, SO TAKE
THE SAME CARE AND ATTENTION WITH THEM.

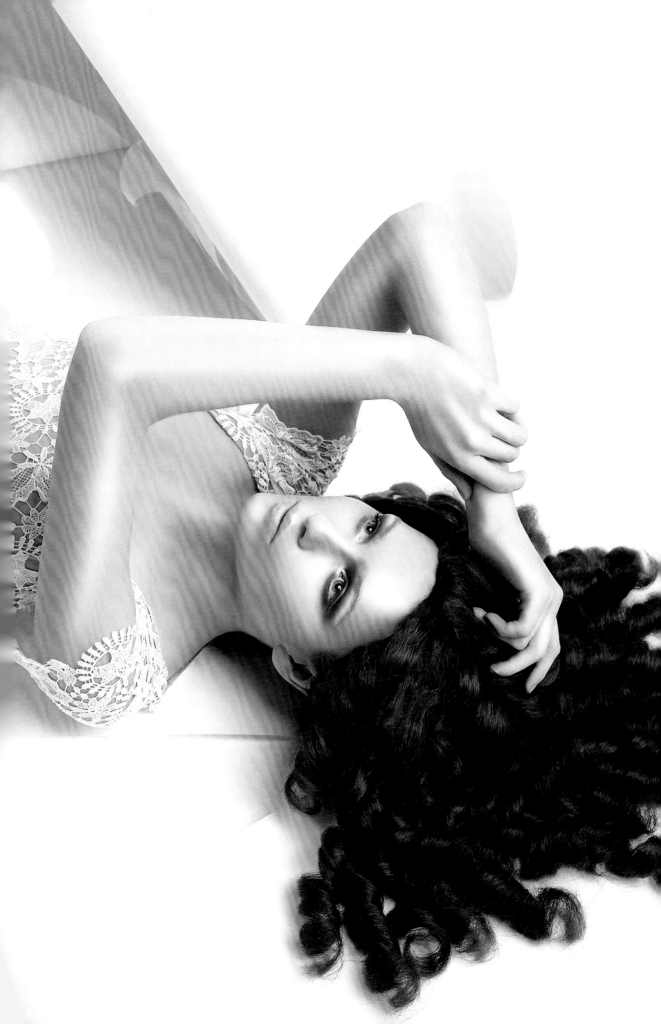

Bare Minimum

Makeup is pared back to its bare essentials with this clean, fresh look. Forgo mascara, pencils, and blush—it's all about a light touch and letting the skin take center stage.

BASE
Charlotte Tilbury Multi-Miracle Glow.
Charlotte Tilbury Charlotte's Magic Cream.
Charlotte Tilbury Light Wonder Foundation in 2 Fair.

CONTOUR
MAC Powder Blush in Taupe.

EYES
MAC Powder Blush in Taupe to shade the creases and underneath the lower lashes.
MAC Eye Kohl in Fascinating on the waterlines.
Becca Shimmering Skin Perfector Pressed Highlighter in Pearl to highlight the inner corners of the eyes and on the eyelids above the pupils.

EYEBROWS
No product; just brush the brows upward and out.

LIPS
Vaseline.

There is such beauty in minimal makeup. Often when I start a strong makeup look and have just finished with the base, sculpting, and highlights, I sit back and think that I would love to stop right there because it just looks so beautiful!

Prior to starting the makeup application, I applied the amazing Charlotte Tilbury Multi-Miracle Glow mask for about ten minutes. I followed this with Charlotte's Magic Cream to really hydrate and plump up the skin. Then I sparingly applied Charlotte Tilbury Light Wonder Foundation in 2 Fair. I continued to set soft highlights using Becca Shimmering Skin Perfector Pressed Highlighter in Pearl above the lips at the Cupid's bow, in the center of the chin, down the nose, and on the inner corners of the eyes. I contoured the cheeks and eyes ever so slightly with MAC Powder Blush in Taupe and added white Eye Kohl from MAC to the waterlines. The lips needed nothing more than a dab of Vaseline. I stopped there: no mascara, no eyebrow pencils, no eyeliner, no blush—just clean and beautiful skin.

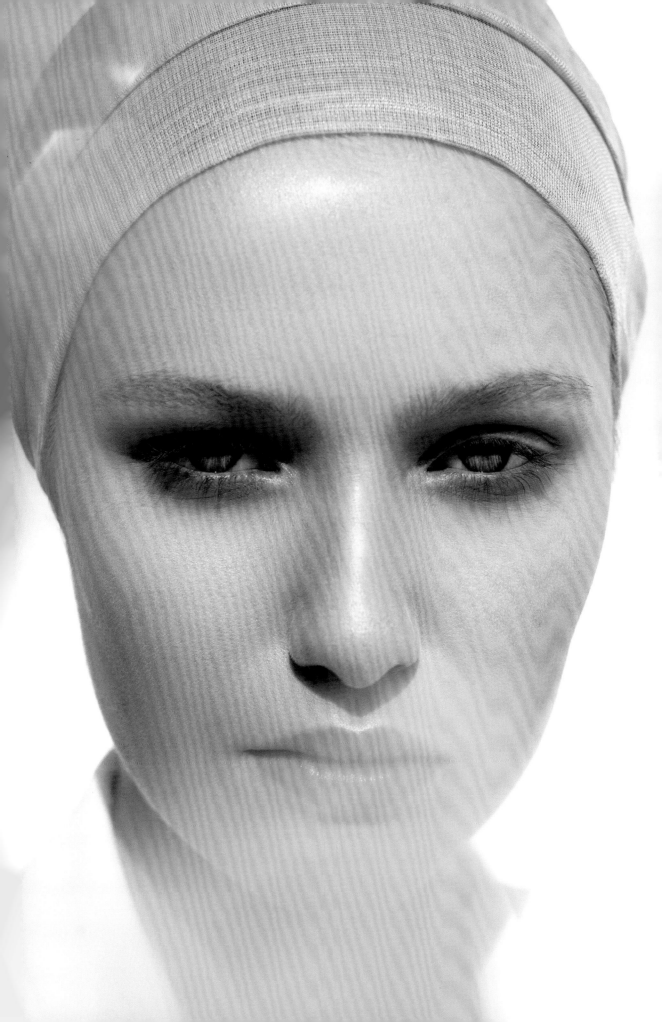

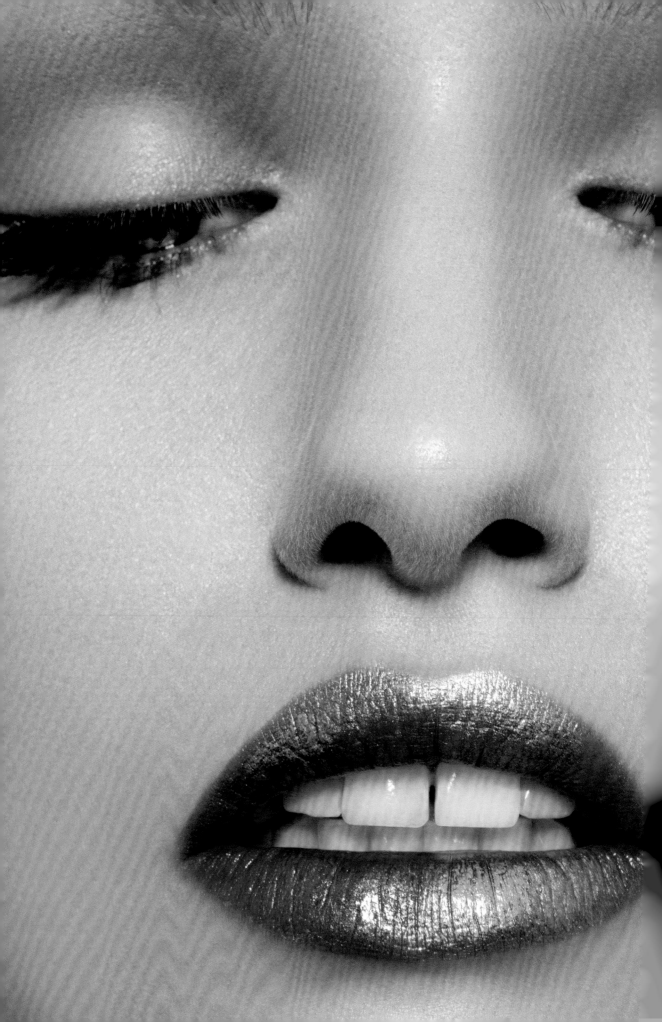

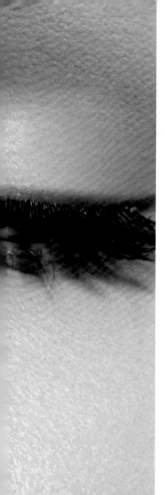

Precious Metal

LIPS GET A MULTICOLORED METALLIC WASH
IN THIS SURPRISING AND BEAUTIFUL LOOK. THE KEY
TO MAKING IT WORK: CLEVER BLENDING AND
KEEPING THE COLOR SLIGHTLY OFFBEAT.

BASE
Very little MAC Pro Full
Coverage foundations in NC15
and NC20 (mixed).
Make Up For Ever HD Powder
to set around the nose,
in the middle of the forehead,
and under the eyes.

HIGHLIGHT
Skin N Nature Cookie Marble
Blusher in 01 Rose.

EYES
MAC Matte Eye Shadow in
Soft Brown blended lightly
over the eyelids with a little
bit more in the creases.
Becca Shimmering Skin
Perfector Pressed Highlighter
in Pearl applied to the inner
corners of the eyes and lightly
over the eyelids.
MAC 30 Lash single lashes
in Medium and Long applied
to the upper lashes.
One coat of black mascara.

LIPS
Kryolan Interferenz
Shimmering Vision Palette.

KRYOLAN'S INTERFERENZ SHIMMERING VISION PALETTE IS A GREAT
PALETTE TO ADD TO YOUR KIT. I USUALLY USE IT TO CREATE REALLY BOLD,
SUPER SHINY METALLIC EYES—AND I LOVE THAT IT ALWAYS PHOTOGRAPHS
SO UNEXPECTEDLY. YOU NEVER REALLY KNOW WHAT IT'S GOING TO LOOK
LIKE UNTIL THE PHOTOGRAPHER HAS FINISHED HIS LIGHTING SETUP AND
STARTS SHOOTING.

HERE, I USED AN ARRAY OF COLORS FROM THE PALETTE. I BEGAN WITH THE
DARK MAGENTA TO DEFINE THE AREAS I WANTED TO KEEP IN A MORE TYPICAL
LIPSTICK COLOR. I THEN ADDED GREEN, LIGHT BLUE, AND FINALLY SILVER AS
A HIGHLIGHT. I LOVE ASYMMETRY, SO I PLACED MY COLORS THIS WAY TO
ADD UNEXPECTEDNESS TO THE IMAGE AND COUNTERACT SOPHIA'S ALMOST
COMPLETELY SYMMETRICAL FACE.

"Before sending your model onto a set, look at whether you can take something off, tweak something, or add something to make it unique and the best it can be. Challenge yourself to find at least one thing that will improve the look."

Toni Malt

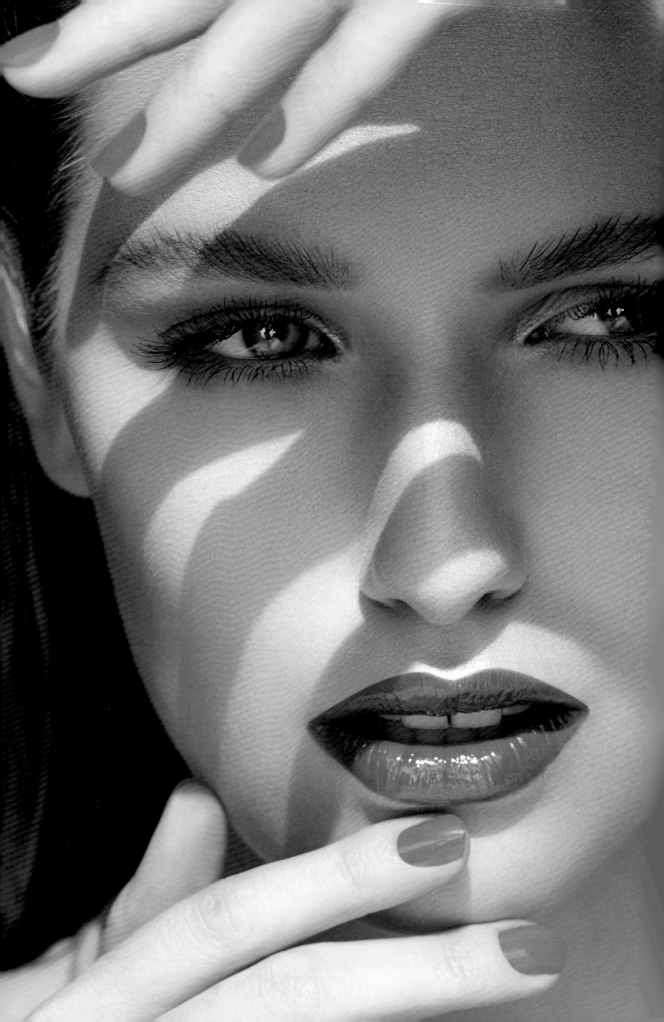

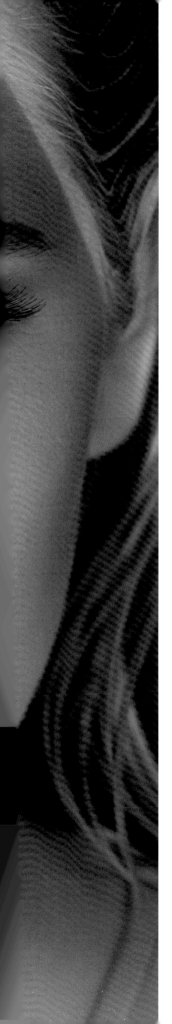

Browlicious

A CLEAN COMPLEXION AND BRUSHED-UP BROWS CREATE
THE IDEAL MAKEUP COMBINATION FOR A HOT-WEATHER SHOOT.
JUST ADD LASHES AND A PERFECT MANICURE.

BASE
Very little MAC Pro Full
Coverage Foundation in NC20.
Make Up For Ever HD Powder
to set.

HIGHLIGHT
Skin N Nature Cookie Marble
Blusher in 01 Rose.

CONTOUR
Illamasqua Powder Blusher
in Disobey.

EYES
MAC Eye Shadow in Taupe
in the creases.
MAC Eye Shadows in Omega
and Vanilla applied to the lids
and the brow bones.
MAC Eye Kohl in Fascinating
on the waterlines.
Becca Shimmering Skin
Perfector Pressed Highlighter
in Pearl applied to the inner
corners of the eyes.
MAC 30 Lash single lashes
in Medium and Long glued
to the upper lashes with DUO
eyelash adhesive.

One coat of black mascara
on top and bottom lashes.

EYEBROWS
Inglot Brow Powders
in 569 and 560.
Redken Forceful 23 Super
Strength Finishing Spray.

LIPS
MAC Lipstick in Morange.
MAC Clear Lipglass.

NAILS
MAC Nail Lacquer in Morange.

BRUSHED-UP, BUSHY EYEBROWS HAVE BEEN A BIG TREND THE PAST FOUR
SEASONS, AND I HOPE IT STAYS THAT WAY, BECAUSE I LOVE THEM.

THERE ARE SEVERAL TECHNIQUES YOU CAN USE TO ACHIEVE THESE GORGEOUS
BROWS. IF YOUR MODEL HAS SOFT EYEBROW HAIRS, IT'S POSSIBLE TO SIMPLY
USE A GOOD BROW GEL. A COLORED BROW GEL WILL BOOST BROW THICK-
NESS EVEN FURTHER; BENEFIT HAS THE GORGEOUS GIMME BROW RANGE.
ALTERNATIVELY, SPRAY A CLEAN MASCARA WAND WITH A STRONG HAIRSPRAY
SUCH AS REDKEN FORCEFUL 23 SUPER STRENGTH FINISHING SPRAY.

IT'S WHAT I USED FOR THIS LOOK; I JUST RAN THE SPRAYED WAND THROUGH
THE EYEBROWS IN AN UPWARD MOTION AND PRESTO, VA-VA-VOOM BROWS.

Color Play

LIPS GET A MULTITONED COLOR HIT WITH THIS BOLD
LOOK. FOR AMAZING PIGMENT PAYOFF, ENLIST HIGH-WATTAGE
LIQUID LIPSTICKS AND OPAQUE CREAMS.

BASE
Very little MAC Pro Full
Coverage Foundation in NC15.
Make Up For Ever HD Powder
to set.

HIGHLIGHT
Skin N Nature Cookie Marble
Blusher in 01 Rose.

CONTOUR
Illamasqua Powder Blusher
in Disobey.

EYES
MAC Eye Shadow in Taupe
in the creases.
MAC Eye Shadows in Omega
and Vanilla applied to the lids
and brow bones.
MAC Eye Kohl in Fascinating
on the waterlines.
Becca Shimmering Skin
Perfector Pressed Highlighter
in Pearl on the inner corners.
MAC 30 Lash single lashes
in Medium and Long glued
to the upper lashes

with DUO eyelash adhesive.
One coat of black mascara
on the top and bottom lashes.

EYEBROWS
Inglot Brow Powders
in 569 and 560.

LIPS
Obsessive Compulsive
Cosmetics Lip Tars in Hoochi,
Demure, and NSFW.
MAC Lipmix in Orange.
MAC Clear Lipglass.

OCC LIP TARS ARE A WONDERFUL PRODUCT. THEY'RE A LIQUID LIPSTICK, SO THEY CAN BE APPLIED LIKE A LIP GLOSS, YET THEY'RE MORE HIGHLY PIGMENTED WITH AMAZING STAYING POWER. THEY ALSO COME IN THE CRAZIEST COLORS, WHICH CAN BE BLENDED TO CREATE CUSTOMIZED HUES.

FOR THE TOP LIP, I MIXED TOGETHER LIP TARS HOOCHI AND DEMURE TO CREATE A PINKISH-PURPLE COLOR. I THEN ADDED DEPTH BY APPLYING NSFW ON THE INNER AND OUTER PART OF THE TOP LIP. ON THE BOTTOM LIP, I USED MAC'S FANTASTIC LIPMIX IN ORANGE. JUST BEFORE SHOOTING, I ADDED HEAPS OF MAC CLEAR LIPGLASS.

WITH SO MUCH PRODUCT ON THE LIPS, BE AWARE OF DRIPS ONCE YOU START SHOOTING. USE A TISSUE, A CLEAN BRUSH, OR A COTTON SWAB TO CLEAN OFF ANY DROPLETS. ALSO, REMIND YOUR MODEL NOT TO RUB HER LIPS TOGETHER OR ALL YOUR COLORS WILL BLEND INTO EACH OTHER.

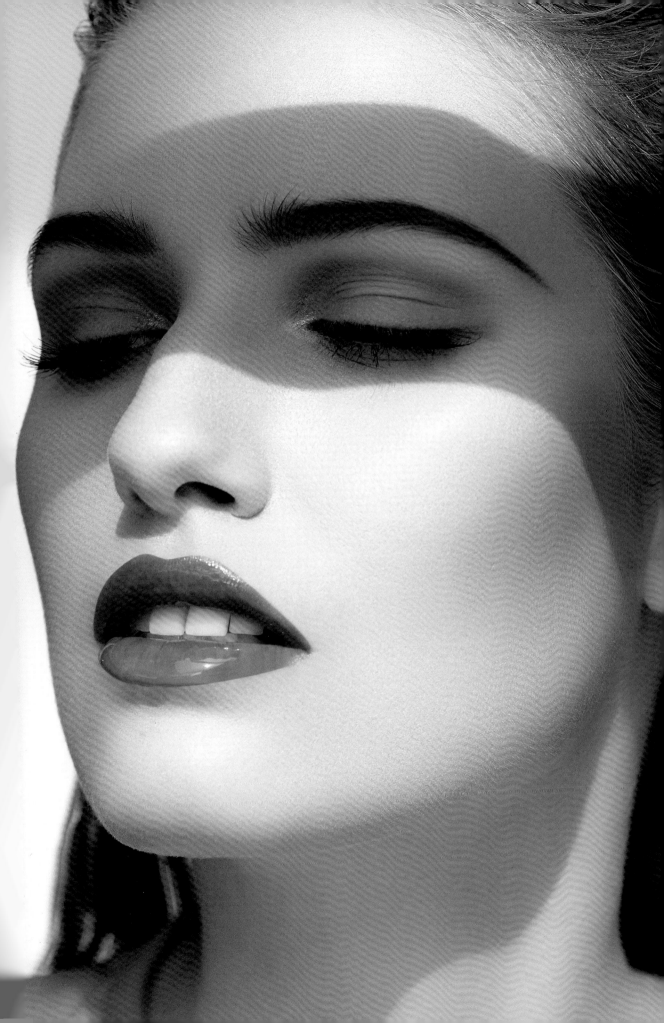

So Glossy

THE HIGH-CLASS NATURE OF THE GLOSSY EYELID MAKES IT HARD TO RESIST. EVEN BETTER, IT'S SUPER EASY TO CREATE.

BASE
Very little MAC Pro Full
Coverage Foundation
in NC15 and NC20.
Make Up For Ever HD Powder
to set.

HIGHLIGHT
Skin N Nature Cookie Marble
Blusher in 01 Rose.

CONTOUR
Illamasqua Powder Blusher
in Disobey.

EYES
MAC Eye Shadow in Taupe
in the creases.
MAC Paint Stick in Genuine
Orange and MAC Clear
Lipglass on the lids.
MAC Eye Kohl in Fascinating
on the waterlines.
Becca Shimmering Skin
Perfector Pressed Highlighter
in Pearl on the inner corners.
MAC 30 Lash single lashes
in Medium and Long glued
to the upper lashes

with DUO eyelash adhesive.
One coat of black mascara
on the top and bottom lashes.

EYEBROWS
Inglot Brow Powders
in 569 and 560.

LIPS
MAC Lip Erase in Dim.

THEY'RE HIGH MAINTENANCE, BUT GLOSSY EYES ALWAYS LOOK SO BEAUTIFUL. I USED MAC PAINT STICK IN GENUINE ORANGE ON THE EYELIDS AND THEN, JUST BEFORE WE STARTED SHOOTING, ADDED MAC CLEAR LIPGLASS ON TOP. IF YOU ARE AIMING FOR A SUBTLER SHINE, USE ELIZABETH ARDEN EIGHT HOUR CREAM INSTEAD OF THE GLOSS. ET VOILÀ, SO SIMPLE!

A GOOD TIP IS TO STAY CLOSE TO YOUR MODEL WHILE SHOOTING. THE CREAMS ON THE EYELIDS WILL CREASE, SO YOU WILL NEED TO KEEP SMOOTHING THEM TO KEEP A PERFECT, SHINY FINISH.

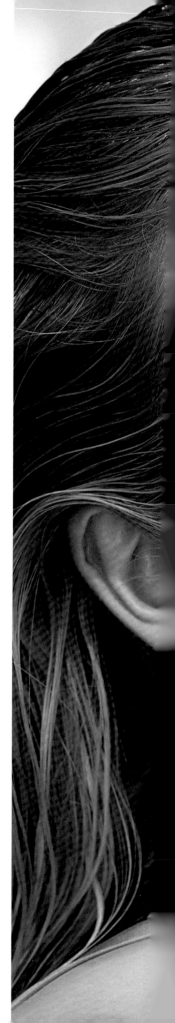

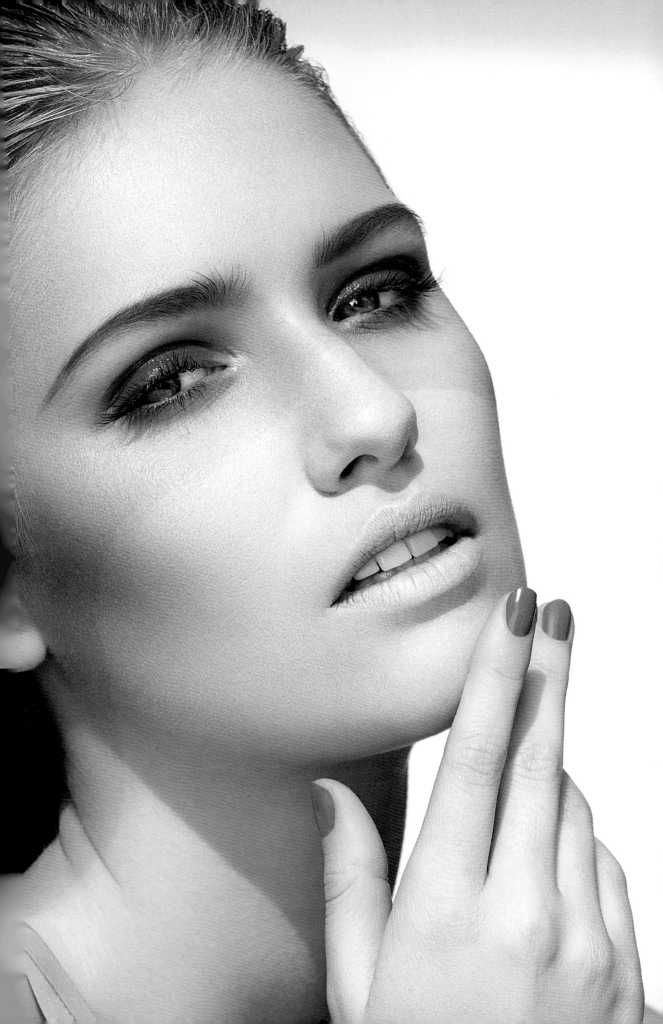

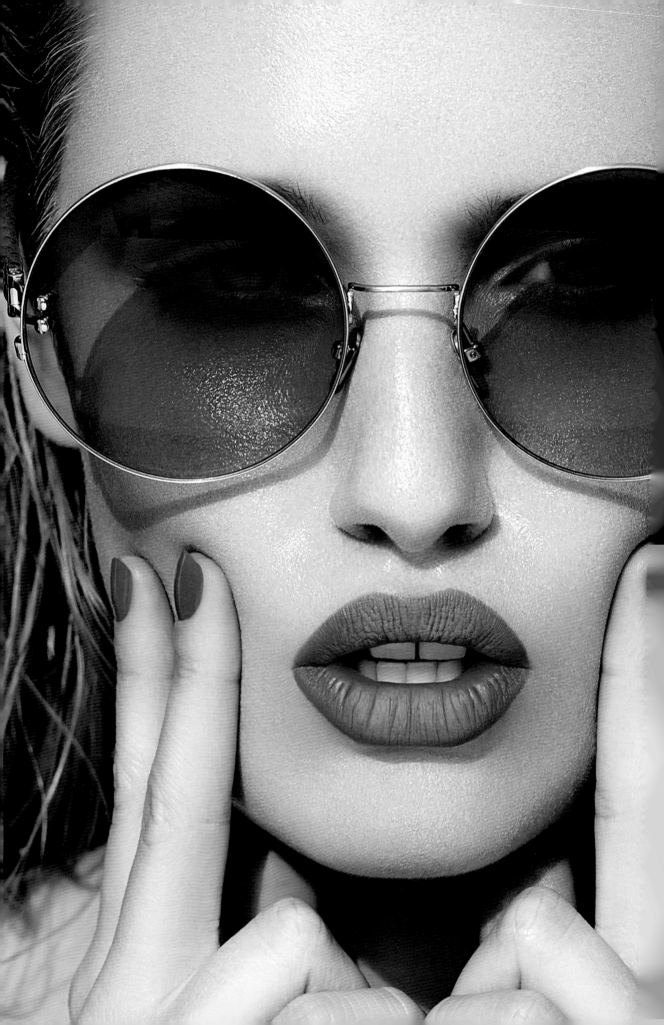

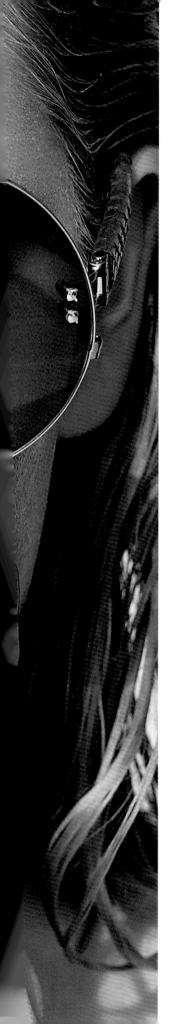

Heat Wave

DON'T JUST STICK TO LIPSTICK AND GLOSS TO TRANSFORM LIPS BOLD AND BRIGHT. A SWEEP OF EYE SHADOW OVER LIPSTICK ADDS A SHOCK OF MATTE ORANGE THAT CRANKS THE HEAT RIGHT UP.

BASE
Very little MAC Pro Full Coverage Foundation in NC20. Elizabeth Arden Eight Hour Cream over foundation.

HIGHLIGHT
Skin N Nature Cookie Marble Blusher in 01 Rose.

CONTOUR
Illamasqua Powder Blusher in Disobey.

EYES
MAC Eye Shadow in Taupe in the creases.
MAC Eye Shadows in Omega and Vanilla applied on the lids and brow bones.
MAC Eye Kohl in Fascinating on the waterlines.
Becca Shimmering Skin Perfector Pressed Highlighter in Pearl on the inner corners.
MAC 30 Lash single lashes in Medium and Long applied to the upper lash lines

with DUO eyelash adhesive. One coat of black mascara on the top and bottom lashes.

EYEBROWS
Inglot Brow Powders in 569 and 560.

LIPS
MAC lipstick in Morange.
Yaby Eye Shadow in es158 Candy Pop.
MAC 239 Eye Shader Brush.

THIS IMAGE IS FROM A BEAUTY EDITORIAL I SHOT WITH SOPHIA FOR *MARIE CLAIRE ARABIA*. WHEN IT WAS PUBLISHED, I GOT SO MANY LOVELY E-MAILS ASKING ME WHAT LIPSTICK I HAD USED TO CREATE THIS BEAUTIFUL MATTE LIP. THE SECRET IS EYE SHADOW. I LOVE MIXING PRODUCTS AND USING THEM TO MULTITASK. I USE BLUSHES AS EYE SHADOWS AND EYE SHADOWS AS CONTOURING POWDERS, AND I OFTEN MAKE LIPSTICKS BY BLENDING EYE SHADOW WITH VASELINE OR CLEAR GLOSS.

SINCE I HAD CREATED A WET LOOK FOR THE SKIN USING ELIZABETH ARDEN EIGHT HOUR CREAM, I WANTED TO EMPHASIZE THE HOT-WEATHER FEELING BY ADDING A CONTRASTING MATTE LIP. I APPLIED MAC LIPSTICK IN MORANGE, THEN I DABBED YABY EYE SHADOW IN ES158 POP CANDY ONTO THE CENTER OF THE LIP USING A MAC 239 EYE SHADER BRUSH. IT'S SUCH A SIMPLE, EFFECTIVE TECHNIQUE!

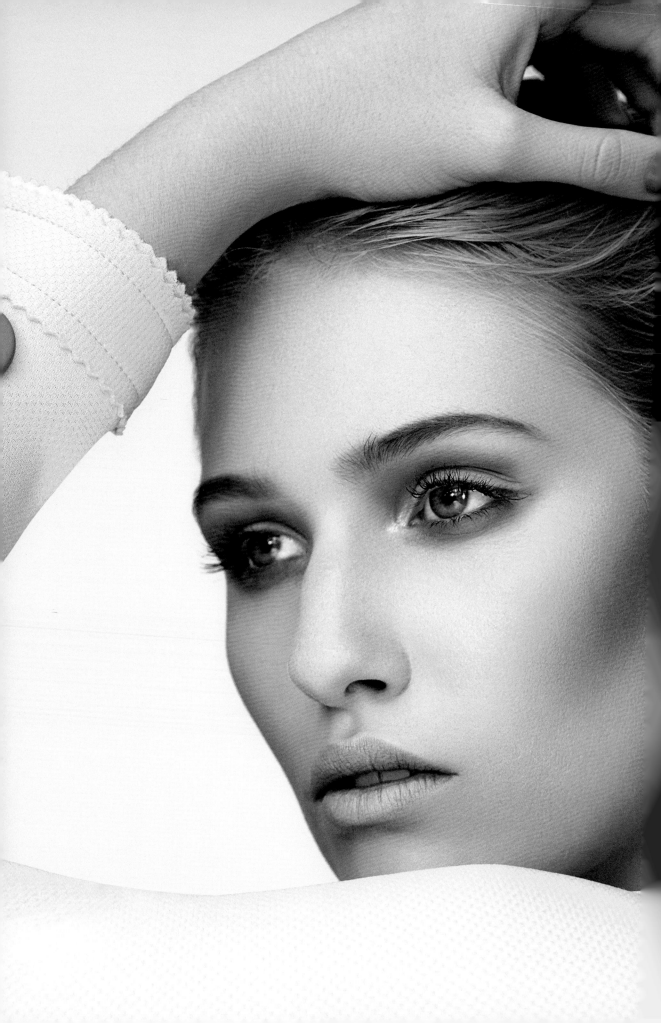

The Big Blend

Contouring gets creative with the help of MAC Paint Sticks. Beautifully blendable with a tactile, skinlike finish, these colorful cream sticks should be a mainstay in every makeup artist's armory.

BASE
MAC Pro Full Coverage Foundation in NC20.

CONTOUR
MAC Paint Stick in Genuine Orange enhanced with MAC Lipmix in Orange.

BLUSH + HIGHLIGHT
MAC Paint Stick in Primary Yellow.

EYES
Bobbi Brown Eye Shadow in Copperplate in the creases. MAC Eye Shadows in Omega and Vanilla applied to the lids and brow bones. MAC Eye Kohl in Fascinating on the waterlines. Becca Shimmering Skin Perfector Pressed Highlighter in Pearl on the inner corners. MAC 30 Lash single lashes in Medium and Long applied to the upper lash lines with DUO eyelash adhesive. One coat of black mascara on the top and bottom lashes.

EYEBROWS
Inglot Brow Powders in 569 and 560.

LIPS
MAC Lip Erase in Dim.

I just love MAC Paint Sticks. This look is simple to do yet has so much impact. I started by contouring below the cheekbones with MAC Paint Stick in Genuine Orange, then used an Illamasqua Blusher Brush to blend in a tiny bit of MAC Lipmix in Orange. For the highlight, I slowly blended in MAC Paint Stick in Primary Yellow with a clean Illamasqua Blusher Brush, starting above the cheekbones and taking the color all the way up into the temples. If there is one product you need to try, MAC Paint Sticks are it!

"Don't automatically assume a look needs black mascara. Brown mascara or even no mascara are equally important options to consider."

Toni Malt

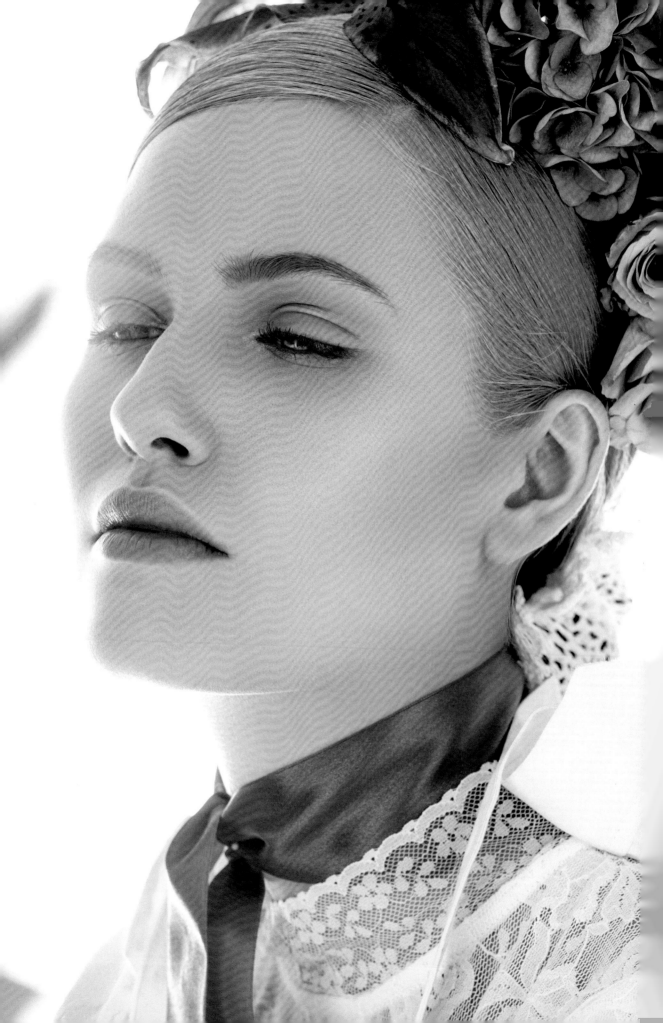

In Full Bloom

ROMANCE IS IN THE AIR WITH THIS BEAUTIFULLY
BLENDED LOOK. SKIN IS PERFECTLY PURE, WHILE
COLOR IS KEPT TO A MINIMUM WITH TONAL SHADES
APPLIED WITH BIG, SOFT BLENDING BRUSHES.

BASE
MAC Pro Full Coverage
Foundations in NC15
and NC20 (mixed).
Armani Luminous Silk Powder
in Ivory to set.

CONTOUR
MAC Cream Color in Fantastic.

EYES
MAC Cream Color Bases in
Luna and Nude as a base.
MAC Matte Eye Shadow in
Soft Brown to subtly enhance.
MAC Eye Kohl in Fascinating
on the waterlines.
One coat of dark brown
mascara.

EYEBROWS
Inglot Brow Powder in 560.

LIPS
MAC Lipstick in Lovelorn
applied with a MAC 239
Eye Shader Brush.
Skip lip liner to maintain
a soft finish.

MY AIM FOR THIS LOOK WAS TO CREATE THE FEELING OF PURITY AND
ROMANCE. BARELY-THERE MAKEUP IS THE KEY TO SUCCESS HERE, SO COLOR
CHOICE AND APPLICATION ARE BOTH REALLY IMPORTANT. THE IDEA IS TO
ACHIEVE PURE VELVET SKIN WITH A ROMANTIC WASH OF COLOR ON THE LIPS,
CHEEKS, AND EYES.

WHEN CHOOSING MY COLORS, I WENT FOR TONAL SHADES AND APPLIED
THEM WITH LARGE, SOFT BLENDING BRUSHES (THE BIGGER, THE BETTER!).
I USED AN ILLAMASQUA BLENDING BRUSH TO BLEND EYE SHADOW INTO THE
EYELIDS. FINALLY, I SOFTLY DABBED THE LIPSTICK ONTO THE LIPS USING A
MAC 239 EYE SHADER BRUSH.

THE AMOUNT OF PRODUCT ON THE BRUSH IS ALSO KEY—LESS IS DEFINITELY
MORE HERE. SLOWLY BUILD COLOR, MAKING SURE ANY EXCESS IS TAPPED
OUT OF THE BRUSH BEFORE APPLYING.

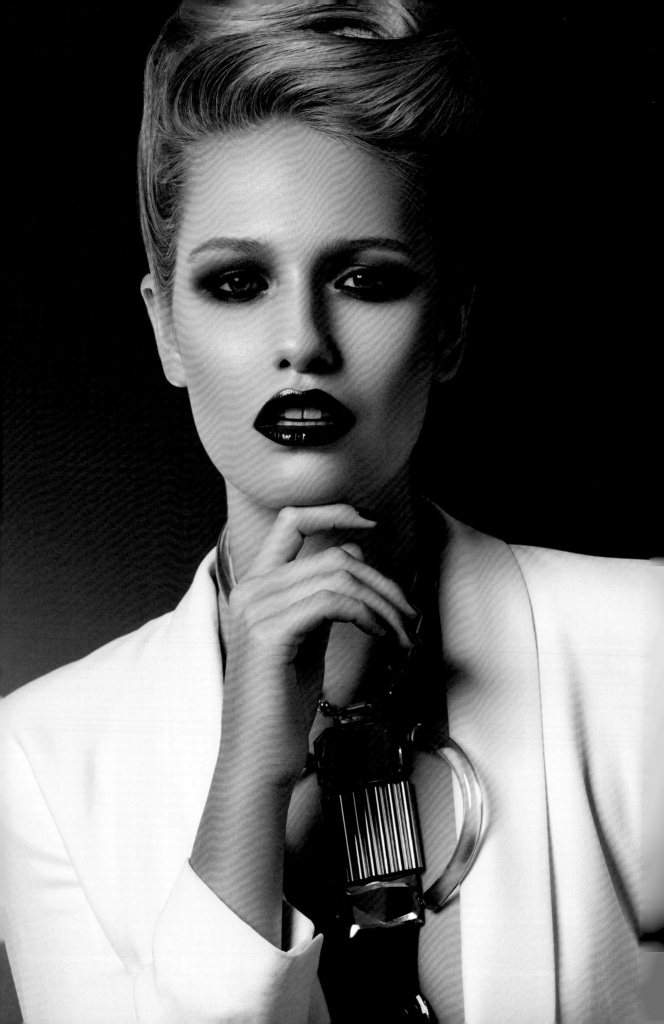

Power Play

THE EXTRAVAGANT ELEGANCE OF THE EARLY 1990s GETS A MODERN-DAY SHOT OF SUPERCHARGED SOPHISTICATION. KEEP THE LOOK FIRMLY IN THIS MILLENNIUM BY PLAYING DOWN THE BROWS AND DITCHING BLUSH.

BASE
MAC Pro Full Coverage Foundation in NC20.
Make Up For Ever HD Powder to set.

CONTOUR
MAC Powder Blush in Taupe.

EYES
Charlotte Tilbury Rock 'n' Kohl Iconic Liquid Eye Pencil in Bedroom Black to tightline the upper waterlines.
Kevyn Aucoin The Essential Eye Shadow N° 110 Blackest Black to rim the eyes.
Yaby Eye Shadows in es491 Sexy Salmon and pp041 Kumquat to create the smoky eyes.
Chanel Illusion D'Ombre in 81 Fantasme.

EYEBROWS
Brushed upward and out.

LIPS
MAC Lip Pencil in Plum.
MAC Lipsticks in Hang Up and Cyber.
MAC Clear Lipglass.

WHILE THIS LOOK IS HIGH ON ELEGANCE AND REMINISCENT OF THE LATE 1980s AND EARLY '90s, IT'S STILL VERY CURRENT. I KEPT IT MODERN BY GIVING THE LIPS AND EYES ALL THE POWER WHILE PLAYING DOWN THE EYEBROWS AND CHEEKS. I LEFT SOPHIA'S BROWS NATURAL AND HER CHEEKS COLOR FREE APART FROM A LITTLE BIT OF MAC POWDER BLUSH IN TAUPE TO CONTOUR UNDER THE CHEEKBONE—HAD I ADDED BLUSH OR ENHANCED SOPHIA'S EYEBROWS, THIS LOOK WOULD VERY QUICKLY HAVE SLIPPED INTO THE '90s.

TO CREATE THE EYES, I TIGHTLINED USING CHARLOTTE TILBURY ROCK 'N' KOHL ICONIC LIQUID EYE PENCIL IN BEDROOM BLACK, THEN RIMMED THE OUTSIDES WITH KEVYN AUCOIN THE ESSENTIAL EYE SHADOW N° 110 BLACKEST BLACK. I FOLLOWED THIS WITH A VERY BLENDED ORANGE-CORAL SMOKY EYE USING A MIX OF YABY EYE SHADOWS IN ES491 SEXY SALMON AND PP041 KUMQUAT. I THEN ADDED MORE DEPTH BY APPLYING MORE OF THE KEVYN AUCOIN THE ESSENTIAL EYE SHADOW CLOSE TO THE LASHES AND THE OUTER CORNERS. TO FINISH OFF, I ADDED CHANEL ILLUSION D'OMBRE IN 81 FANTASME TO THE INNER CORNERS OF THE EYES.

TO ADD EXTRA GLAMOUR, I CREATED A DARK, SULTRY LIPSTICK BY MIXING MAC LIPSTICKS IN HANG UP AND CYBER TOGETHER, THEN FINISHED WITH A LITTLE MAC CLEAR LIPGLASS ON TOP.

Float Away with Me

GETTING MAKEUP TO STAY FLAWLESS DURING DIFFICULT SHOOTS CALLS FOR MAKEUP WITH SERIOUS STAYING POWER. THIS BRONZED LOOK HAD TO WITHSTAND HOT CAMERA LIGHTS AND LONG PERIODS IN WATER: NINETY MINUTES LATER AND IT'S STILL LIKE NEW.

BASE
MAC Pro Full Coverage Foundation in NW30. Illamasqua Blusher Brush.

CONTOUR
Tom Ford Shade and Illuminate in 01 and 02—dark shades mixed.

EYES
Tom Ford Shade and Illuminate in 01 as a base to contour the eyes in the creases and underneath.
Maybelline Eye Studio Color Tattoo 24HR Cream Gel Shadow in 35 On and On Bronze to enhance.
Maybelline Eye Studio Color Tattoo 24HR Cream Gel Shadow in 70 Barely Branded to set highlights on the brow bones, eyelids, and inner corners.
MAC Eye Kohl in Fascinating on the waterlines.
MAC 30 Lash single lashes in Medium and Long.
Black waterproof mascara.

LIPS
MAC Lipstick in Morange.
MAC Clear Lipglass.

SKIN
Scott Barnes Body Bling Shimmering Body Lotion in Platinum.

BEING BASED IN DUBAI, A COUNTRY WHERE TEMPERATURES REGULARLY REACH 100°F AND ABOVE, I OFTEN NEED TO ENLIST WATERPROOF MAKEUP THAT CAN WITHSTAND HEAT AND PERSPIRATION WHEN I'M WORKING ON LOCATION. EMOLLIENT FOUNDATIONS AND EYE SHADOWS CAN TAKE SOME GETTING USED TO, BUT IF YOU PICK YOUR PRODUCTS WISELY, THEY'RE NOTHING TO BE AFRAID OF. THE BEST ADVICE I CAN GIVE IS TO CHOOSE CREAMS OVER POWDERS.

THE FOUNDATION I USED FOR THIS LOOK WAS MAC PRO FULL COVERAGE FOUNDATION IN NW30—A SLIGHTLY DARKER SHADE THAN I'D NORMALLY USE ON SOPHIA—TO CREATE THE BASE TO A BEAUTIFUL TAN. I THEN CONTOURED THE CHEEKS AND EYES BY MIXING THE DARKER SHADE OF BOTH 01 AND 02 OF TOM FORD SHADE AND ILLUMINATE COMPACTS. IT'S A WONDERFUL PRODUCT THAT REALLY STAYS PUT—ALTERNATIVELY, THE VERY CLEVER MULTITASKING MAC CREAM COLOR BASE COULD ALSO BE USED. TO ENHANCE THE EYES FURTHER, I USED MAYBELLINE'S BEAUTIFUL COLLECTION OF LONG-LASTING CREAM EYE SHADOWS CALLED EYE STUDIO COLOR TATTOO 24HR CREAM GEL SHADOW. I USED SHADE 35 ON AND ON BRONZE TO ENHANCE THE SHADING I'D ALREADY DONE IN THE CREASES AND UNDERNEATH THE EYES, THEN USED 70 BARELY BRANDED TO HIGHLIGHT THE EYELIDS AND INNER CORNERS.

IT TOOK US AN HOUR AND A HALF TO GET THESE TWO SHOTS, AND TRUST ME, WITH ALL THAT TIME SOPHIA SPENT IN THE BATHTUB, THERE WAS PLENTY OF WATER WASHING OVER HER FACE. BUT REMARKABLY, THE MAKEUP STAYED PUT AS IF NOTHING HAD HAPPENED. WHEN I DID HAVE TO DRY OFF SPOTS OF WATER, I JUST ABSORBED THE WATER BY GENTLY PRESSING A COTTON PAD AND THEN STIPPLING MY ILLAMASQUA BLUSHER BRUSH—WHICH I USED FOR MY FOUNDATION APPLICATION—OVER THE AREA TO REESTABLISH THE SKIN TEXTURE.

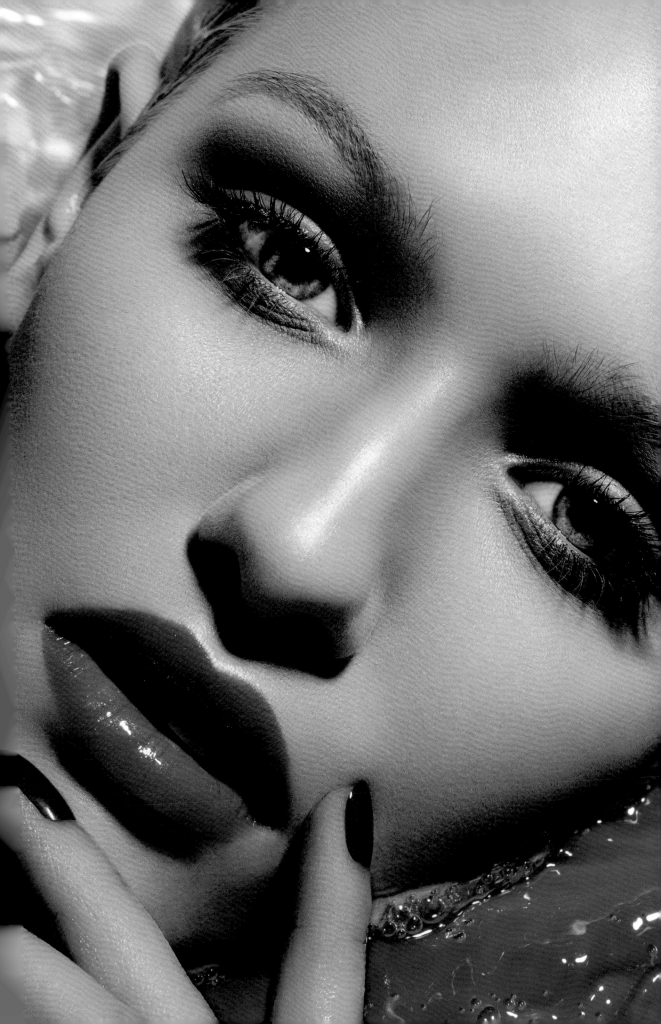

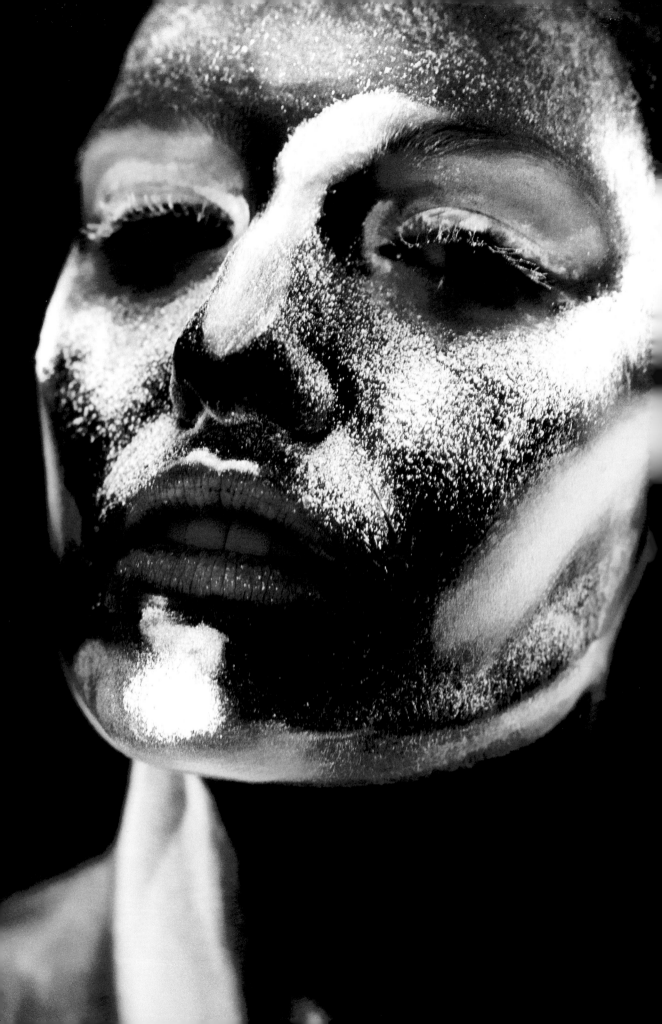

Shadow Play

MAKEUP GOES FREESTYLE WITH THE NEW-AGE WAVE
OF UV-SENSITIVE PRODUCTS HITTING THE MARKET.
GLOW IN THE DARK IS NO LONGER SIMPLY CHILD'S PLAY.

PRIMER
Two layers of Illamasqua
Satin Primer.

SKIN
Make Up For Ever Fluo Night
Black Light Pigments in
27 White, 28 Fuchsia, 32 Blue,
and 33 Green.

I USED MAKE UP FOR EVER'S CLEVER UV LIGHT-SENSITIVE FLUO NIGHT BLACK LIGHT PIGMENTS TO CREATE THIS LOOK. THERE ARE A FEW OF THESE TYPES OF LIGHT-SENSITIVE COLORS HITTING THE MARKET, BUT I'D NEVER WORKED WITH THEM BEFORE, SO THIS WAS A FIRST FOR ME. IT WAS REALLY FUN, BUT AT THE SAME TIME, I HAD TO PAY CLOSE ATTENTION TO WHAT I WAS DOING. I FOUND THE TRICK WAS TO IMAGINE THAT I WAS TRANSFORMING A BLACK ONE-DIMENSIONAL FACE INTO A THREE-DIMENSIONAL FACE THROUGH PIGMENT PLACEMENT.

TO DO THIS, I CONSIDERED WHICH AREAS OF A FACE USUALLY GET HIGHLIGHTED BY LIGHT (THE BRIDGE OF THE NOSE, THE CUPID'S BOW, THE MIDDLE OF THE CHIN, THE TOPS OF THE CHEEKBONES, THE TEMPLES, THE INNER CORNERS OF THE EYES, THE MIDDLE OF EACH EYELID, AND THE MIDDLE OF THE FOREHEAD) AND WHICH ARE CONTOURED (THE JAWLINE, THE HOLLOWS OF THE CHEEKS, THE CREASES OF THE EYES, THE SIDES OF THE FOREHEAD, ABOVE THE TEMPLES, AND RIGHT UNDERNEATH THE MIDDLE OF THE BOTTOM LIP). I TRIED TO SPRINKLE MOST OF THE HIGHLIGHTED AREAS WITH UV PIGMENT AND ACCENTUATE MOST OF THE CONTOURED AREAS WITH BRUSHSTROKES.

I ALSO PAINTED A LITTLE UV PIGMENT ACROSS THE LIPS TO GIVE THE MOUTH DEFINITION; IF I'D LEFT THEM BLANK, THERE WOULD HAVE BEEN A BLACK HOLE WHERE THE LIPS ARE MEANT TO BE. THAT'S ACTUALLY A GOOD WAY TO THINK OF THIS METHOD OF MAKEUP: WHEREVER YOU DO NOT PUT PIGMENT, YOU HAVE BLACKNESS, SO IF YOU PUT NO UV PIGMENT ON THE BRIDGE OF THE NOSE, YOU WILL HAVE NO NOSE. THE SAME GOES FOR THE NECK AND SHOULDERS: IF YOU IGNORE THEM, YOU WILL HAVE A FLOATING HEAD WITHOUT A BODY.

THE ONE THING THAT DIDN'T SHOW UP IN A CONVINCING WAY WAS THE COLORS. UNDER UV LIGHT, THE FINISH WAS JUST A WASH OF BLUE, BLACK, WHITE, AND YELLOW, SO WE TRANSFORMED THE IMAGE IN POSTPRODUCTION INTO THIS BLUE-TINTED BLACK AND WHITE VERSION. I THINK THE RESULT IS EERILY BEAUTIFUL.

Sparkle and Shine

SOMETIMES IT'S THE OUTFIT THAT SPARKS THE CREATIVE FIRE.
THIS MINXY VIBE WAS INSPIRED BY A SEASONAL HIT: MARC JACOBS'S
SPRING-SUMMER 2013 EMBELLISHED MICKEY MOUSE SWEATER. PRRRRR...

BASE
MAC Pro Full Coverage
Foundation in NC15
and NC20 mixed.
Make Up For Ever HD Powder
to lightly set the T-zone.

CONTOUR
Illamasqua Powder Blusher
in Disobey.

HIGHLIGHT
Laura Mercier Loose Shimmer
Powder in Star Dust.

EYES
Charlotte Tilbury Rock 'n' Kohl
Iconic Liquid Eye Pencil in
Bedroom Black to line the eyes.
Kevyn Aucoin The Essential
Eye Shadow N° 110 Blackest
Black to enhance.
Make Up For Ever Extra Large
Size Glitter in NO2 Silver.
DUO eyelash adhesive in Clear.
Eylure Girls Aloud Lashes
in Nicola. Black mascara on
the top and bottom lashes.

LIPS
MAC Lip Pencil in Redd.
MAC Lipsticks in Ruby
Woo and So Chaud mixed.
MAC Clear Lipglass.

THIS LOOK WAS A LOT OF FUN TO DO—I HARDLY RECOGNIZE OUR BEAUTIFUL MODEL SOPHIA! IT'S VERY SEXY MAKEUP WITH BLACK FELINE EYES AND MIGHTY RED LIPS, SO TO GET IT TO WORK WITH THE CLOTHES—AND IN PARTICULAR, THE MARC JACOBS EMBELLISHED MICKEY MOUSE SWEATER—IT NEEDS TO HAVE A FUN ELEMENT. TO ACHIEVE THIS, I DECIDED TO ADD THE OVERSIZE SILVER GLITTER EYE EMBELLISHMENT, A LOOK INSPIRED BY THE AMAZING NEW YORK-BASED MAKEUP ARTIST LOTTIE.

TO CREATE THE FELINE EYES, I USED CHARLOTTE TILBURY ROCK 'N' KOHL ICONIC LIQUID EYE PENCIL IN BEDROOM BLACK TO RIM AROUND THEM AND EXTEND A FLICK AT THE OUTER CORNERS. I THEN ADDED KEVYN AUCOIN THE ESSENTIAL EYE SHADOW N° 110 BLACKEST BLACK OVER THE TOP OF THE LINER TO ACHIEVE SUPER-MATTE, BLACK EYES—A BEAUTIFUL CONTRAST FOR THE SILVER GLITTER. TO CREATE THE GLITTER EMBELLISHMENT, I SPREAD A VERY THIN LAYER OF DUO EYELASH ADHESIVE IN CLEAR OVER THE EYE AREA, STOPPING ABOVE THE EYEBROWS BEFORE GENTLY PRESSING THE MAKE UP FOR EVER EXTRA LARGE SIZE GLITTER IN NO2 SILVER ONTO THE PREPARED AREA. THE PRO ONLY LINE AT MAKE UP FOR EVER HAS SUCH A GREAT SELECTION OF FANTASTIC GLITTERS, SO DO MAKE TIME TO VISIT ONE OF THEIR STORES—IT'S A REAL TREASURE TROVE!

I WOULD NORMALLY USE KRYOLAN GLITTER GEL TO APPLY GLITTER, BUT FOR THIS LOOK, I OPTED FOR THE STRONGER DUO EYELASH ADHESIVE. AS I KNEW THE HAIR WOULD BE RUBBING AGAINST THESE SUPER-LARGE GLITTERS, I WANTED TO MAKE SURE THEY STAYED PUT THE ENTIRE SHOOT.

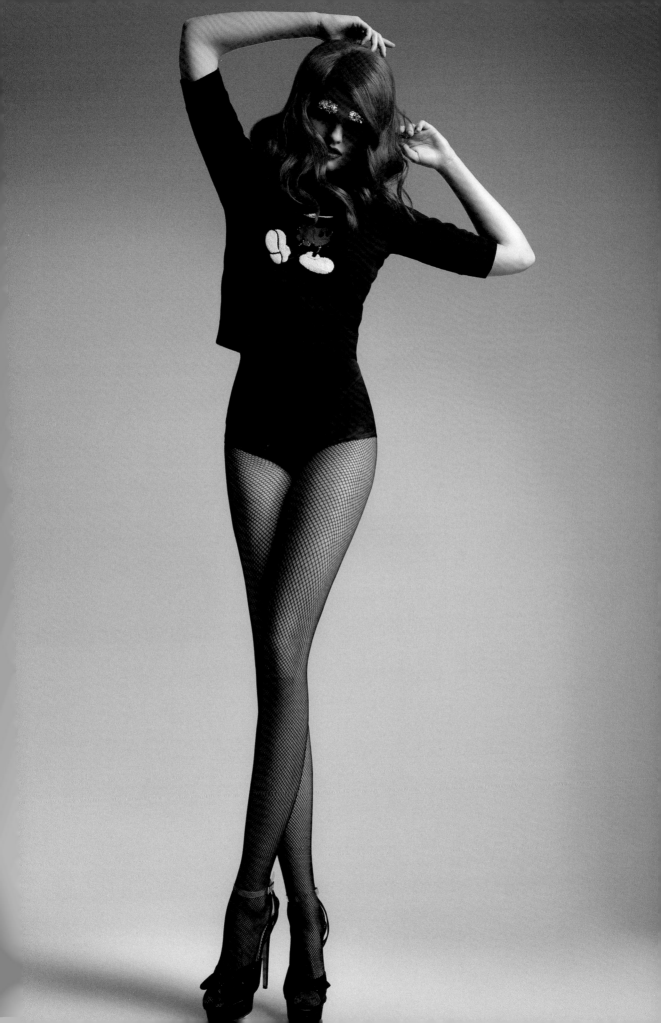

"Deconstruct a look
to experiment with
thinking outside of the
box of traditional makeup.
This will enable you to
create new unique looks."

Toni Malt

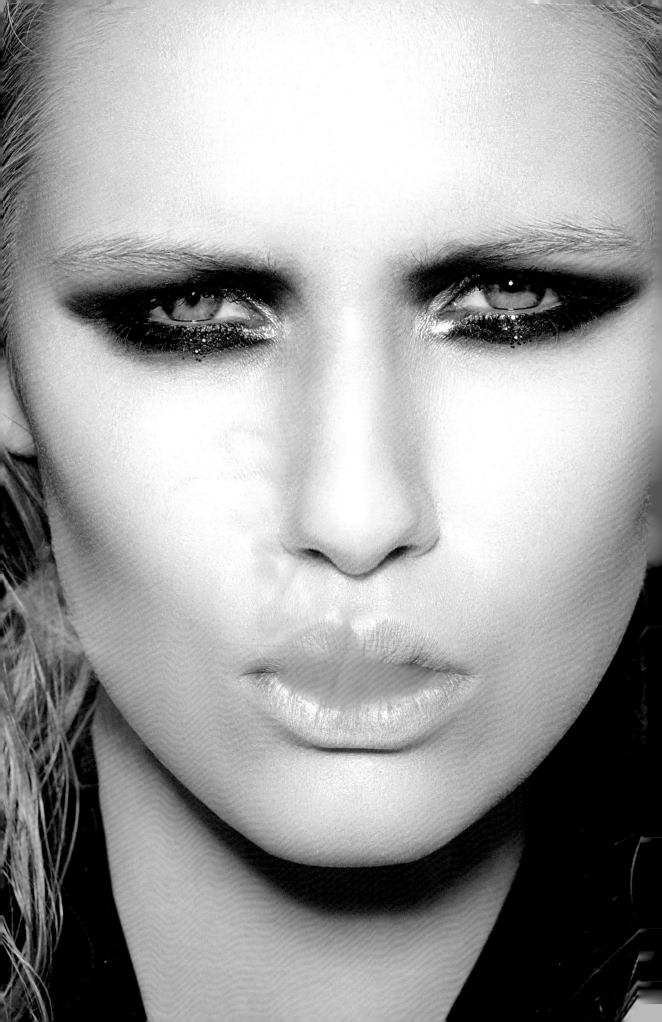

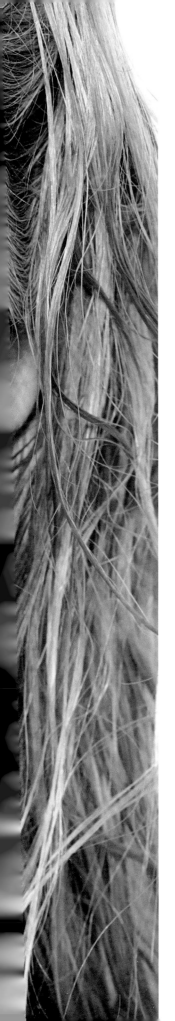

Wild One

The way to nailing the rocker-chic look is dark, not-too-perfect eyes; neutral lips; and plenty of attitude. The meek need not apply.

BASE
Charlotte Tilbury Light Wonder Foundation in 2 Fair.
Make Up For Ever HD Powder over the T-zone.

CONTOUR
Charlotte Tilbury Cheek to Chic Swish & Pop Blusher in First Love.

EYES
Kevyn Aucoin The Essential Eye Shadow Nº110 Blackest Black.
MAC Eye Kohl in Fascinating.
Illamasqua Liquid Metal in Solstice on the inner corners.
Make Up For Ever Medium Size Glitters in N48 Black.
Kryolan Clear Glitter Gel.
Black mascara on the top and bottom lashes.
MAC Eye Shader 239 Brush and MAC 217 Blending Brush.

EYEBROWS
A small amount of MAC Pro Full Coverage Foundation in NC15 combed through the brows with a mascara wand to lighten.

LIPS
MAC Lip Erase in Pale dabbed onto the lips with the fingers.

HIGHLIGHT
Laura Mercier Star Dust Loose Setting Powder.

I love a great rock chick-inspired look—it's just so full of attitude. The smoky eye shape here gives Sophia this stern, skeptical expression. She looks like she's frowning, but she isn't—it's all makeup.

Flawless skin and strong, slightly imperfect eyes are key in achieving a great rocker-chic look. I actually went slightly lighter on the foundation here to emphasize the darkness and strength of the eye makeup—the barely-there eyebrows and natural-looking lips also helped with this. For the eyes, I applied Kevyn Aucoin The Essential Eye Shadow Nº110 Blackest Black using MAC brushes 239 and 217. I started near the bridge of the nose, then took the black eye shadow up into the start of the eyebrows before sweeping it across the eyelids and beyond the outer lashes. Finally, I added lots of black eye shadow underneath the lower lashes, pulling it out to the sides, where I connected it with the eye shadow on the eyelids. I left the inner corners free of black eye shadow, instead highlighting them—slightly imperfectly—using Illamasqua Liquid Metal in Solstice and a touch of MAC Eye Kohl in Fascinating. I applied black mascara to the top and bottom lashes, then finished off with a tiny bit of black glitter underneath the pupils, which I applied with Kryolan Clear Glitter Gel.

69

On the Edge

This modern look demands more than just brave makeup application—it requires model participation. Sophia applied her own eyeliner and lip cream so she could truly own it.

PREP
Charlotte Tilbury
Multi-Miracle Glow.
Charlotte Tilbury
Charlotte's Magic Cream.
Dior Glow Maximizer Primer.

BASE
Charlotte Tilbury Light Wonder
Foundation in 2 Fair.

CONTOUR
Tom Ford Shade & Illuminate
Intensity One.

HIGHLIGHT
Tom Ford Shade & Illuminate
Intensity One.

EYES
Tom Ford Shade & Illuminate
Intensity One to lightly shade
the creases.
MAC Eye Kohl in Smolder
to tightline the eyelashes.
Black mascara on the top
and bottom lashes.

LIPS
Color 512 G from Kryolan
Shimmering Vision Palette
mixed with MAC Pro Mixing
Medium Matte.

Edgy looks can be challenging. Living and working mainly in Dubai and Asia, my briefs are usually based around the fine-tuning of modern glamour, so this super contemporary look, although simple, is not a makeup look I often get asked for.

I felt that the only way I could tackle this brief for green lipstick was to create a makeup look for a super-confident girl—one who is cool enough to pull off something as out-there as green lipstick. I felt the key to making it work was to minimize my use of product and give the skin a cool "no-makeup" look.

Achieving a great no-makeup look is all down to preparation. The skin needs to be as smooth as possible, so I asked Sophia to exfoliate her face the night before. Then, on the day of the shoot, I started with a ten-minute face mask, followed by Charlotte Tilbury's beautifully nourishing Charlotte's Magic Cream. Over this I applied an illuminating primer from Dior. The result was glowing, healthy skin. I then enhanced the skin with the tiniest amount of foundation to create a beautifully modern and three-dimensional complexion. Less is more here, so I steered clear of setting powder.

I chose to use only cream products, so the Tom Ford Shade & Illuminate came in handy to both contour and highlight the cheeks and eyes ever so slightly. I asked Sophia to tightline her eyes herself by lining her top and bottom waterlines with MAC Eye Kohl in Smolder. She also applied the Kryolan Color 512 G to her lips—I simply perfected the shape afterward and added MAC Pro Mixing Medium Matte to tone down the shine. I wanted Sophia to own this difficult look, so she needed to be part of the creation.

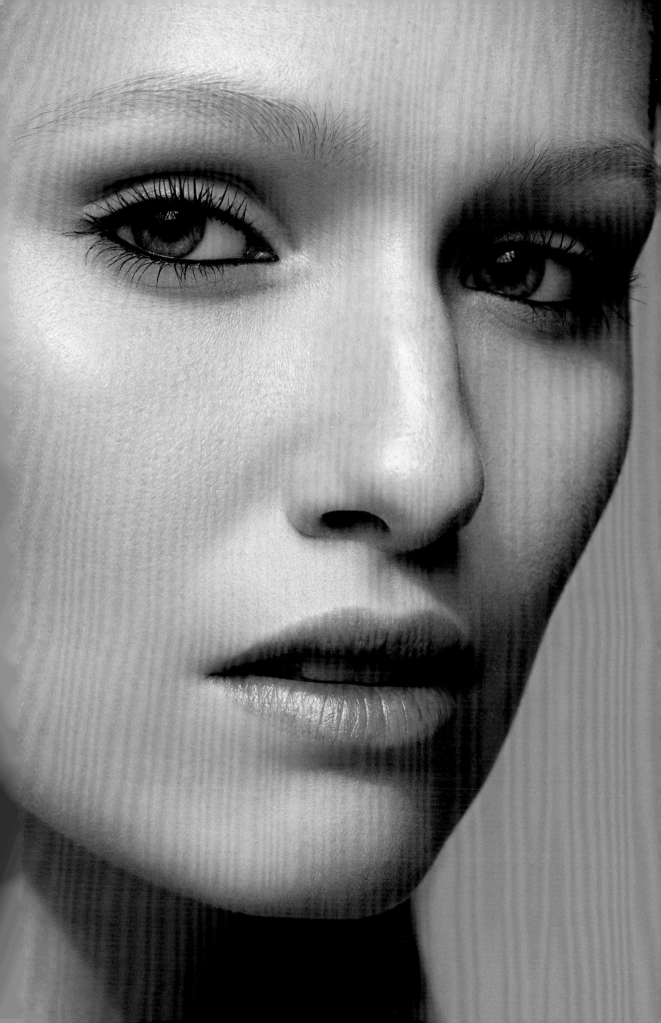

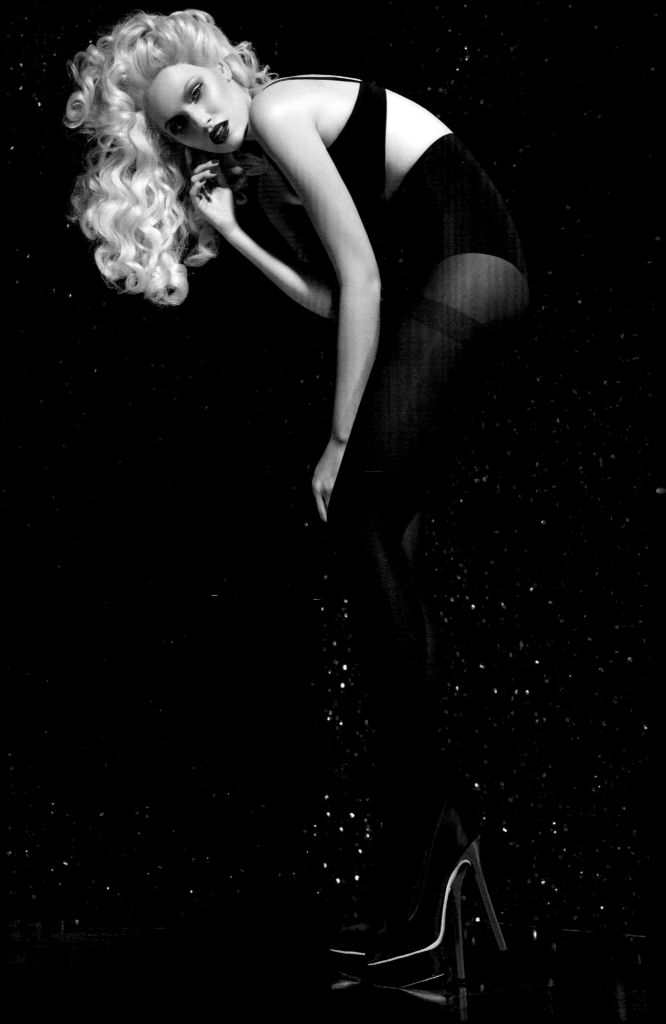

Bombshell Red

The 1950s American pinup gets a modern makeover. Lips go screen-siren red, eyes are almond sleek, and hair is big and platinum. The key to keeping it firmly in the now: clean sculpted skin and barely-there brows.

BASE
Charlotte Tilbury Light Wonder Foundation in 2 Fair.
MAC Pro Full Coverage Foundation in NC15 on the center of the face.
Make Up For Ever HD Powder to set.

CONTOUR
MAC Powder Blush in Taupe.

LIPS
MAC Lip Pencil in Redd to outline and fill.
Lancôme L'Absolu Rouge Lipstick in 132 Caprice.
Make Up For Ever HD Powder.
Inglot 4SS brush to apply powder.
MAC Clear Lipglass applied generously.

EYEBROWS
MAC Pro Full Coverage Foundation in NC15 brushed through (use a disposable mascara wand) to soften the look of the brows.
Avoid caking by starting at the outer edge of the brows and working the mascara wand against the growth of the hair.
Work a clean mascara wand against the hairs if you get too much product on the brows.

EYES
Yaby Eye Shadows in Baby Grizzly and Royal Brown (from the Yaby Dramatically Neutral Palette) to shape the eyes.
Illamasqua Pure Pigment in Breathe to highlight the eyelids and inner corners.
MAC Eye Kohl in Fascinating on the waterlines.
MAC 30 Lash single lashes in Medium and Long.
Black mascara.

The main focus of this modern Marilyn Monroe look is the fire engine-red glossy lips. I'm always excited when I get to do super-red, glossy lips because they look amazing on just about everyone. Red lips also photograph beautifully, so they're exciting from an editorial point of view as well.

I always start with the lips when I'm creating a bold statement lip because I find it helps me balance the lips with the eyes. I generally like a full roundish upper lip, so I used MAC Lip Pencil in Redd to create a really soft, round Cupid's bow. I then filled in the lips with pencil to create a base for the lipstick and applied one coat of the incredible Lancôme L'Absolu Rouge Lipstick in 132 Caprice. It's a really vibrant true red and must be my favorite lipstick in the whole wide world. I blotted the lips with a single sheet of tissue before dabbing some Make Up For Ever HD Powder over them using an Inglot 4SS brush. I followed with a second coat of lipstick, then, just before shooting, I applied several coats of MAC Clear Lipglass. So many layers of gloss can cause drips on the lower lip, so have a tissue or cotton swab on standby.

To create the soft, smoky effect on the eyes, I used Yaby Eye Shadow in Baby Grizzly ES575, leaving the eyelids lighter than the rest of the eye area. I then enhanced the creases and below the lower lash lines with Royal Brown ES562. I added MAC Eye Kohl in Fascinating to the waterlines and brightened the inner corners of the eyes and the eyelids just above the pupil with Illamasqua Pure Pigment in Breathe. To help visually extend the eyes outward, I curled the lashes and applied one coat of black mascara before adding MAC 30 Lash single lashes in Medium to the top lashes and a single MAC 30 Lash in Long at the very end.

California Dreaming

INSPIRED BY THE OVER-THE-TOP, STREET-SMART STYLE OF SOUTHERN CALIFORNIA'S LATINAS, THIS LOOK IS ALL ABOUT THE TATTOO-LIKE BROWS AND LINED NEUTRAL LIPS. JUST ADD PLENTY OF ATTITUDE.

BASE
MAC Pro Full Coverage Foundation in NW20.
Make Up For Ever HD Powder to set.

CONTOUR
Bobbi Brown Eye Shadow in Tan to contour the hollows of the cheeks.

HIGHLIGHT
Skin N Nature Cookie Marble Blusher in 01 Rose.

EYES
Bobbi Brown Eye Shadow in Tan to contour the eyes in the creases and below the lashes.
MAC Fluidline in Blacktrack to create a thin line on the top lashes.
Girls Aloud Lashes by Eylure in Nicola.
Illamasqua Pure Pigment in Breathe on the inner corners of the eyes.

EYEBROWS
Elmer's All Purpose School Glue Stick to glue the outer parts of the eyebrows flat.
MAC Eye Brows pencils in Stud and Spiked to enhance and extend brow shape.

LIPS
MAC Lip Erase in Dim.
MAC Lip Pencil in Stone.

I LOVE LATINAS. THEY HAVE SUCH STREET-SMART ATTITUDE. THEY MIX TOO MUCH MAKEUP AND OVERDONE HAIR WITH SUPER-RELAXED CLOTHES—CONVERSE, KHAKIS, AND TANK TOPS ARE THE UNIFORM—AND SOMEHOW IT ALL JUST WORKS.

THE KEY TO ACHIEVING THIS LATIN-INSPIRED LOOK IS TO FOCUS ON THE EYEBROWS AND THE LIPS; YOU WANT TO ADD STRENGTH AND POWER TO THE FACE WHILE KEEPING THE LOOK BEAUTIFUL. BEFORE APPLYING FOUNDATION, I BRUSHED DOWN THE OUTER HALVES OF SOPHIA'S BROWS WITH A CLEAN MASCARA WAND, THEN GLUED THE HAIRS IN THE DIRECTION OF GROWTH USING AN ELMER'S ALL PURPOSE SCHOOL GLUE STICK. IT CAN TAKE BETWEEN TWO AND FOUR COATS BEFORE THE BROWS LIE FLAT.

AFTER FOUNDATION, I USED MAC EYE BROWS PENCILS IN STUD AND SPIKED TO STRENGTHEN THE SHAPE OF THE UNGLUED PARTS OF THE BROWS AND REDRAW THE OUTER HALVES INTO BEAUTIFUL FULL ARCHES. I USE TWO SHADES OF BROW PENCIL BECAUSE I FIND IT HELPS CREATE A REALISTIC THREE-DIMENSIONAL ARCH.

I CREATED THE LIPS BY DABBING ON A LITTLE BIT OF MAC LIP ERASE IN DIM WITH MY FINGER, THEN HIGHLIGHTING THE CUPID'S BOW WITH ILLAMASQUA PURE PIGMENT IN BREATHE. TO ACHIEVE THAT SIGNATURE LATINA VIBE, I LINED THE LIPS WITH A BROWN LIP PENCIL BY MAC.

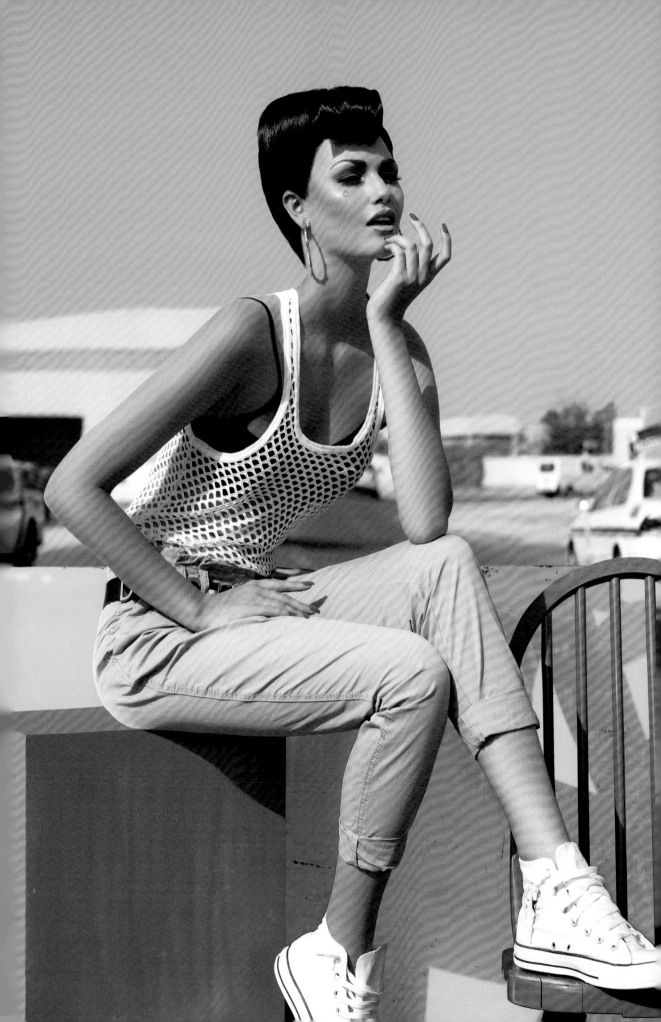

Dream Weaver

INSPIRED BY THE FEARLESS AND MAGICAL WORK OF MAKEUP ARTIST YASMIN HEINZ, THIS ETHEREAL LOOK IS FULL OF UNPREDICTABLE INTRIGUE.

BASE
MAC Pro Full Coverage
Foundation in NC20.
Make Up For Ever HD Powder
to set.

CONTOUR
MAC Pro Paint Sticks in Marine
Ultra and Hi-Def Cyan.

EYES
MAC Eye Shadows in Omega
and Charcoal Brown (mixed).
MAC Eye Lashes in 33.
Black mascara on the top lashes.
Illamasqua Pure Pigment in
Breathe on the inner corners.

I LOVE DOING THIS KIND OF MAKEUP—ITS BEAUTY IS SO UNPREDICTABLE. THIS LOOK IS A NOD TO THE REBELLIOUSLY BEAUTIFUL WORK OF MAKEUP ARTIST YASMIN HEINZ. HER BRAVERY WITH TECHNIQUE AND HER COMMITMENT TO HER ART IS TRULY INSPIRING AND MAKES HER ONE OF THE MOST SOUGHT-AFTER ARTISTS OF OUR TIME. I HAVE BEEN FORTUNATE ENOUGH TO ATTEND ONE OF YASMIN'S MASTER CLASSES, AND SHE REALLY TAUGHT ME SO MUCH ABOUT BEING BRAVE WITH MY MAKEUP.

I BEGAN BY GLUING DOWN THE EYEBROWS WITH ELMER'S ALL PURPOSE SCHOOL GLUE STICK. OF ALL THE BROW-FLATTENING TECHNIQUES, I FIND THIS IS THE BEST. I BRUSH THE EYEBROWS WITH A CLEAN MASCARA WAND, THEN SIMPLY SLIDE THE GLUE STICK OVER THE HAIRS. I LET THE GLUE DRY, THEN APPLY ADDITIONAL COATS UNTIL THE EYEBROWS ARE GLUED FLAT—THIS TAKES BETWEEN TWO AND FOUR COATS. AFTER GLUING THE BROWS, I STIPPLED FOUNDATION OVER THEM WITH A MAC 217 BRUSH, THEN SET WITH LOTS AND LOTS OF MAKE UP FOR EVER HD POWDER APPLIED WITH A POWDER PUFF.

I USED MAC EYE SHADOWS IN OMEGA AND CHARCOAL BROWN TO ADD A STRONG CONTOUR TO THE EYES, THEN ADDED A PAIR OF MAC EYE LASHES IN 33 AND A COAT OF BLACK MASCARA. TO ACHIEVE THE BEAUTIFUL SHAPE OF THE NEW EYEBROWS, I CAREFULLY MAPPED OUT THE START, HIGH POINT, AND END OF EACH BROW WITH DOTS OF MAC'S WHITE EYE KOHL. TO DRAW THE BLACK LINE, I USED A SIGMA E17 BRUSH AND MAC FLUIDLINE IN BLACKTRACK. TRY TO DRAW YOUR EYEBROWS IN ONE FLUID LINE; YOU CAN FIX UP ANY MISTAKES AFTERWARD WITH A COTTON SWAB DIPPED IN A HEAVY MOISTURIZER.

EYEBROWS
Elmer's All Purpose School
Glue Stick.
MAC Pro Full Coverage
Foundation in NC20.
MAC 217 Blending Brush.
MAC Eye Kohl in Fascinating.
MAC Fluidline in Blacktrack
to create new eyebrows.
Sigma E17 brush.
Make Up For Ever HD Powder
to set.

LIPS
MAC Lipstick in Lovelorn applied
with a MAC 239 brush to create
a soft feel.

SPECKLES
MAC Pro Chromacakes in Pure
White, Primary Yellow, and Cyan.
DIY paintbrushes.

For the beautiful blue contour, I used an Illamasqua Blusher Brush to apply MAC Pro Paint Sticks in Marine Ultra mixed with Hi-Def Cyan. Then it was time for the fun part—the speckling!

MAC Pro Chromacakes are highly pigmented solid-color cakes that activate with water. After I had activated all three colors, I dipped ordinary DIY paintbrushes into the three different pigments, then speckled Sophia's face by running my fingers along the brush. (Make sure your model's eyes are closed at all times throughout this process.) The closer you are to the face, the more control you have over where the color will sprinkle. I followed the principles of highlighting and contour for this look by adding cyan sprinkles where I would naturally shade the face, and yellow and white where I would normally highlight. I also speckled the neck, hair, and ears to keep the face balanced. This is messy, so before you begin, make sure your model is wearing protective clothing and the floor is covered.

The look is more polished if the eyelashes are free of any colored paint, so a good tip is to check the eyelashes for splashes of color. Simply paint over any spots using an eyeliner brush filled with black mascara.

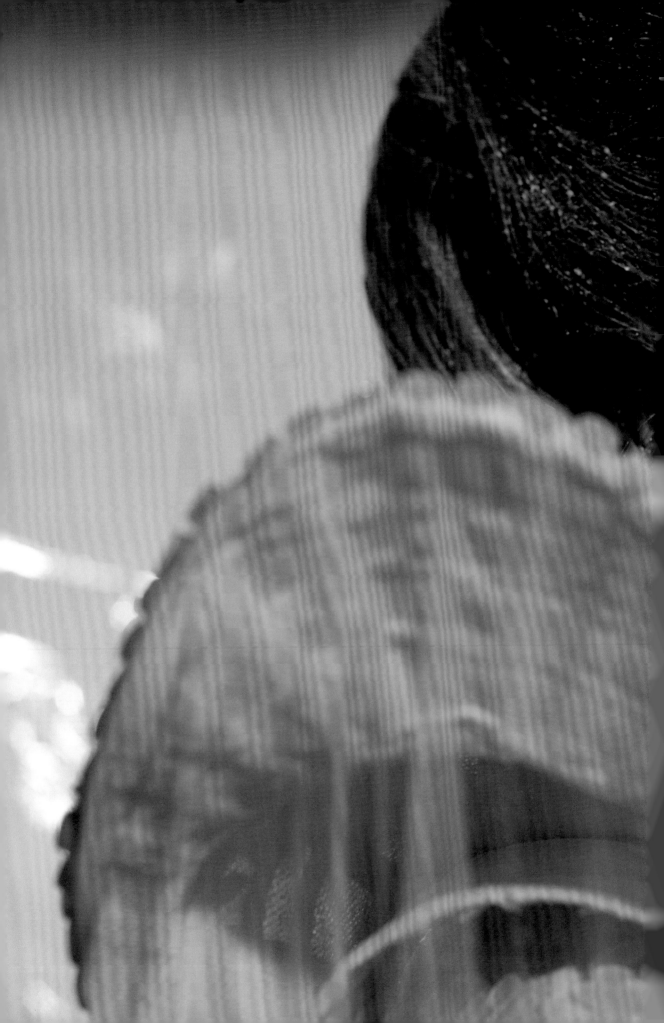

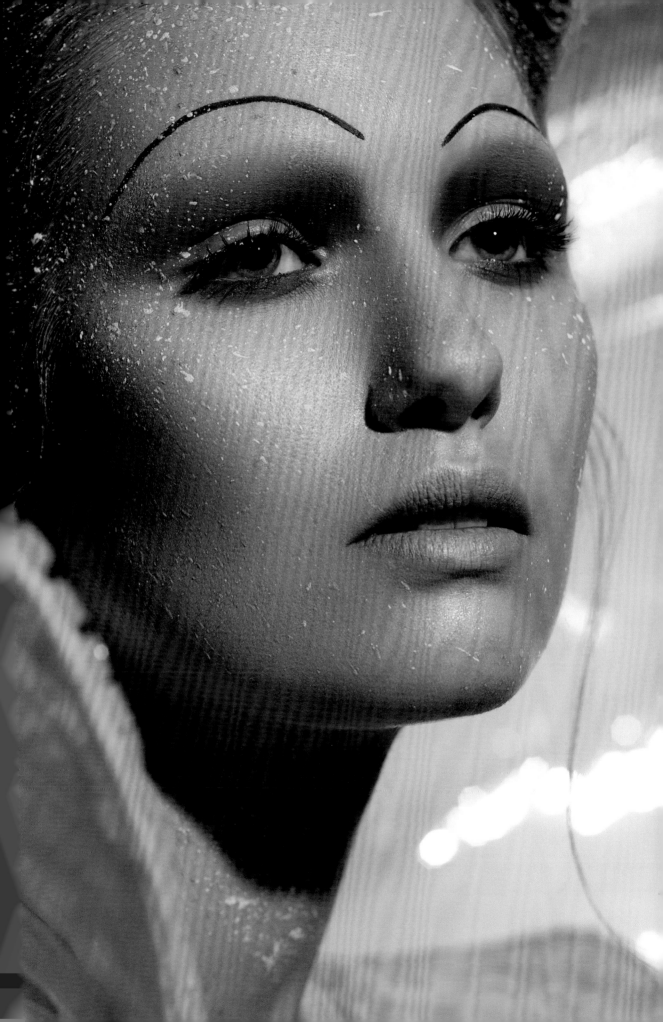

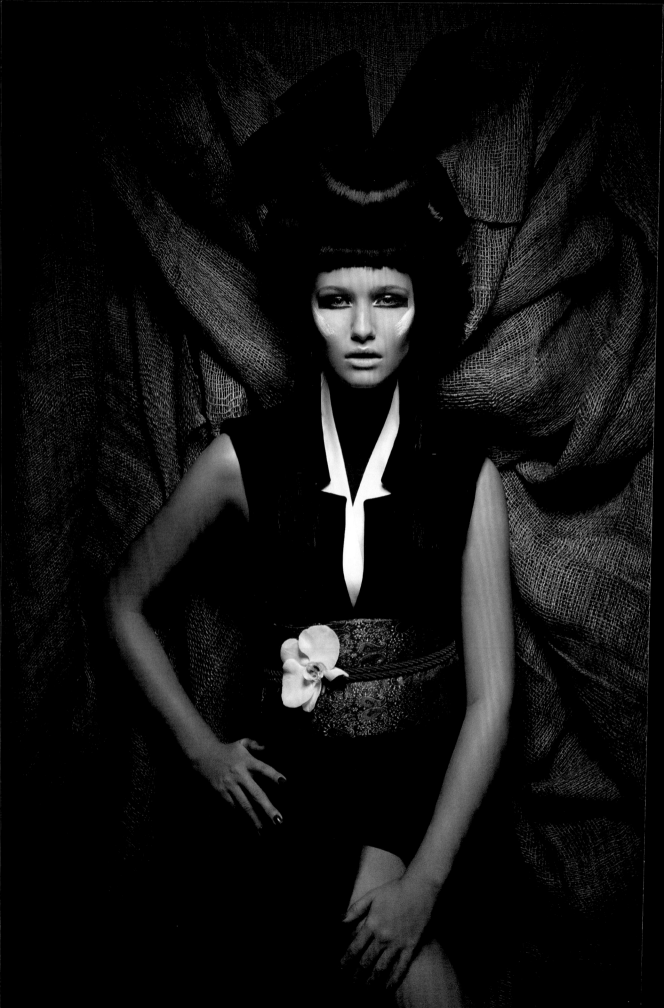

Japanese Love Story

The world of the geisha is an enduring source of inspiration for fashion editorial. Here the geisha gets a fiercely modern update with warriorlike paint and bold calligraphy-inspired highlights.

BASE
MAC Pro Full Coverage in NC20.
Make Up For Ever HD Powder
to set.

HIGHLIGHT
MAC Pro Paint Stick in Pure
White applied with a 1-inch
industrial hard-bristle brush.

CONTOUR
MAC Powder Blush in Taupe.

EYES
MAC Powder Blush in Taupe
to contour the creases.
MAC Pro Paint Stick in Basic Red
to create a rectangular shape
around the eyes.
Yaby Eye Shadow in es287
Hibiscus (from the Yaby
Something Bright palette)
to set.
Yaby Eye Shadow in pp080
First Snow (Something Bright
palette) to add a strong
highlight above the pupils
and inner corners.

LIPS
Brush lips lightly with whatever
foundation is left on the
foundation brush.
A small amount of MAC Lipstick
in Lovelorn dabbed in the center
of the lips for barely-there color.

NECK
Four coats of Illamasqua
Satin Matte Primer applied
on the neck.
MAC Chromacake in Basic Red
applied with a MAC 128 Split
Fiber Cheek Brush.

I really enjoy the process of researching, so I love receiving briefs that include ethnic or cultural inspirations. The Japanese geisha is a recurring theme for editorial fashion shoots, so I've had many opportunities to delve into this beautiful makeup look.

For this look, I wanted to create a more modern take on the traditional geisha. There is actually a wide variety of geisha makeup, so I was keen to demonstrate that a geisha is not only defined by a bee-stung lip and white skin; it's possible to omit these elements and still retain that geisha feel.

The eyes, the highlight on the cheekbones, and the red neck are all key in this look. In Japanese culture, the nape has a sensual meaning, and traditionally, many geishas left their napes unpainted to bare their vulnerability. Because I wanted my geisha to be a super-strong, almost warriorlike figure, I painted her entire neck red, disguising all skin and vulnerability. To unite the red neck with the rest of the face, I painted red rectangular shapes around the eyes and finished off with a dab of pink on the center of the lips.

I decided to channel the beauty of old Japanese calligraphy by painting bold white highlights down the cheekbones. To do this, I used a 1-inch-wide DIY brush with stiff bristles and MAC Pro Paint Stick in Pure White. This idea was inspired by the stunning Chanel Métiers d'Art Pre-Fall 2014 show, where they brushed gold lines onto the temples.

I love this image, but I feel so sorry for Sophia every time I look at it because of the pain she went through. The three real-hair wigs and many hairpieces we'd put in her hair made her head so heavy that my lovely stylist Lisa had to hold Sophia's head from behind while I finished the makeup as quickly as I could. Poor Sophia was completely exhausted before we had even started shooting, just from trying to hold her head up. Clearly, it's not easy being a geisha!

Future Shock

PORCELAIN WHITE SKIN WITH A HIT OF NEON PINK GIVES THIS LOOK
A FUTURISTIC FEEL THAT'S OUT OF THIS WORLD. DON'T BE AFRAID TO BLEND
PRODUCTS: THIS LOOK IS A LESSON IN UTILIZING WHAT'S AT HAND.

BASE
MAC Pro Full Coverage
Foundations in NC15
and White (mixed) stippled
with Illamasqua Blusher Brush.
Make Up For Ever HD Powder
pressed into the skin with
a powder puff to set.

BODY
MAC Pro Full Coverage
Foundations in NC15 and White
(mixed) applied to the hands,
legs, and stomach.
Make Up For Ever HD Powder
to set.

CONTOUR
Flormar Neon Eyeshadow
in N104 Pink applied with
a MAC 116 Blush Brush.

EYES
Yaby Eye Shadow in pp005
Pink Tourmaline (from the Yaby
World of Pearl Paint palette)
on the eyelids.
Illamasqua Pure Pigment in
Breathe on the inner corners.
Maybelline Great Lash Clear
Mascara for Lash and Brow
mixed with Flormar Neon
Eyeshadow in N2014 Pink.
MAC 7 Lash.
MAC 205 Mascara Fan Brush.

EYEBROWS
A small amount of MAC Pro Full
Coverage Foundation in NC15
brushed through the eyebrows
with a mascara wand.

LIPS
Vaseline to moisturize the lips.
MAC Pro Full Coverage
Foundation in NC15.

WHAT MAKES THIS LOOK SO POWERFUL IS ITS SIMPLICITY: WHITE SKIN WITH
LOTS OF NEON PINK MASCARA AND NEON PINK BLUSH APPLIED ALL THE WAY
INTO THE TEMPLES.

I LOVE BLENDING PRODUCTS TO CREATE MY OWN MAKEUP. HERE, I MADE
MY OWN NEON PINK MASCARA BY MIXING MAYBELLINE GREAT LASH CLEAR
MASCARA FOR LASH AND BROW WITH FLORMAR NEON EYESHADOW IN N104
PINK. I SIMPLY SCOOPED OUT THE MASCARA AND SCRAPPED OFF SOME OF THE
EYE SHADOW WITH A SPATULA, THEN BLENDED THEM BOTH UNTIL I HAD AN
EVENLY COLORED PASTE. TO CREATE THE EYES, I GLUED THE MAC 7 LASHES
ON TOP OF SOPHIA'S NATURAL LASHES AND APPLIED FOUR COATS OF PINK
MASCARA, BOTH ON TOP AND UNDERNEATH THE LASHES, USING A MAC 205
MASCARA FAN BRUSH. TO ADD MAXIMUM IMPACT, WHILE THE MASCARA WAS
STILL WET, I APPLIED LOOSE PINK PIGMENT—AGAIN, SCRAPED OFF FROM
THE FLORMAR NEON EYESHADOW—ON THE TOP AND BOTTOM LASHES WITH A
MAC 228 MINI SHADER BRUSH.

I ALSO USED THE NEON EYE SHADOW AS A BLUSH. TO CREATE AN ETHEREAL,
OTHERWORLDLY FEEL, I SWEPT THE BEAUTIFUL COLOR ACROSS THE SIDES OF
THE FACE, INTO THE TEMPLES, AND ONTO THE EYES. THE LIPS NEEDED TO BE
RECESSIVE TO MAKE THE EYES STAND OUT, SO I APPLIED VASELINE TO ADD
MOISTURE, THEN APPLIED MAC PRO FULL COVERAGE FOUNDATION IN NC15.
KEEP IN MIND THAT THIS TECHNIQUE DOES DRY OUT THE LIPS AND WILL
ONLY LAST ONE SHOT. IF YOU WANT TO CREATE THESE LIPS FOR A FULL DAY
OF SHOOTING, BE PREPARED TO REMOVE THE PRODUCT, REMOISTURIZE, AND
REAPPLY AT EACH LOOK CHANGE.

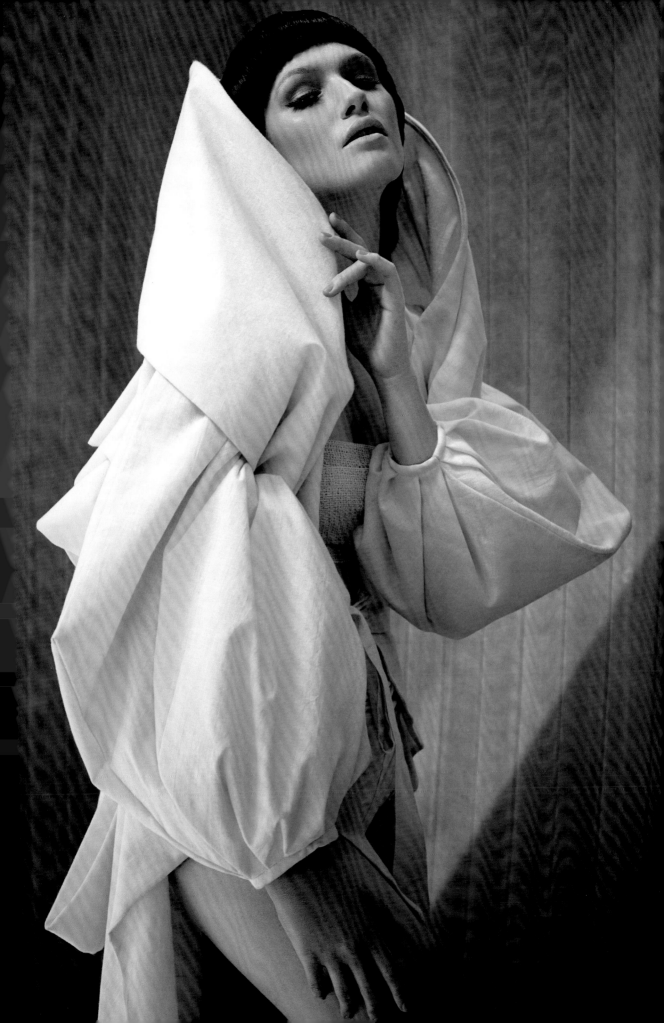

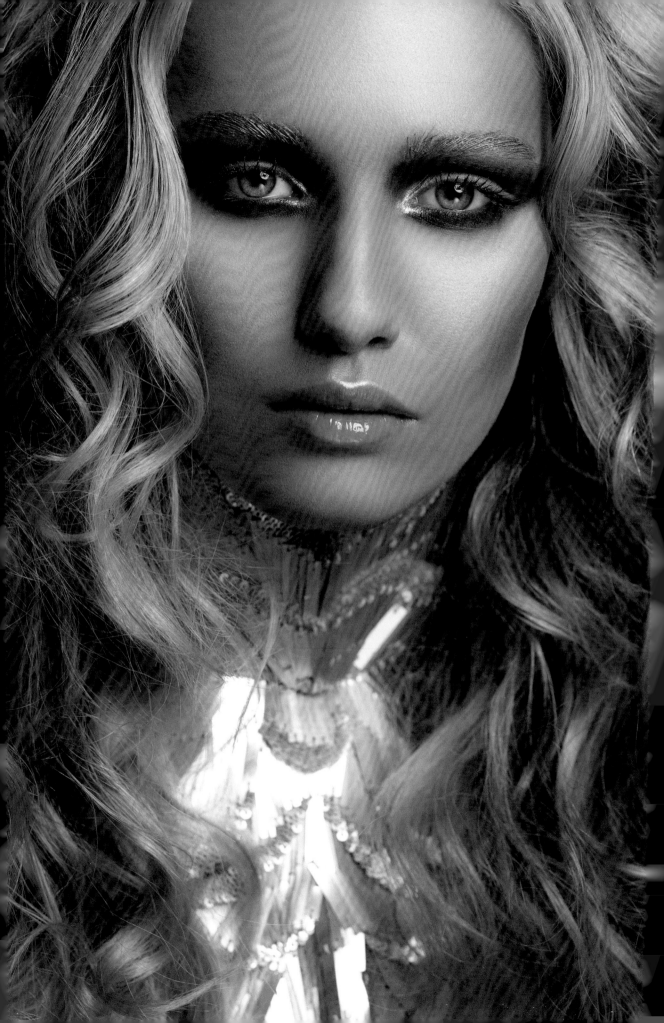

Glamazon Gold

Decadently bronzed skin, fierce eyes, and gold-flecked eyebrows crank the glamour stakes right up.

BASE
MAC Pro Full Coverage
Foundation in NW30.
A small amount of Make
Up For Ever HD Powder to set.

HIGHLIGHT
Laura Mercier Star Dust Loose
Setting Powder in Star Dust.

CONTOUR
Illamasqua Bronzer in Writhe.

EYES
Illamasqua Bronzer in Writhe
on the eyelids.
Kevyn Aucoin The Essential Eye
Shadow in N° 110 Blackest Black
to contour the eyes from the
creases up toward the brows
as well as underneath
the lower lashes.
Illamasqua Liquid Metal
in Solstice to highlight
the inner corners.
Lots of MAC 3 Lash single
lashes in Medium and Long
glued to the top lashes.
One coat of black mascara
on the top and bottom lashes.

EYEBROWS
Fekkai Hi-Lights Hair Mascara
in Gold.

LIPS
MAC Lip Pencil in Subculture
applied all over the lips.
Dior Addict Lip Maximizer.
Illamasqua Liquid Metal in
Solstice on the Cupid's bow.

I originally designed this look for the cover of *Velvet* magazine in 2011. The brief was loosely based on Roberto Cavalli's beautiful ultra-tanned girls that season.

I started by turning Sophia a beautiful bronze (she was thrilled with her new golden tan!) using a darker shade of foundation than I would normally use on her skin tone and Illamasqua Bronzer. Once I'd finished the smoky eye makeup, I added six layers of Fekkai Hi-Lights Hair Mascara in Gold through Sophia's eyebrows. I really wanted to build up the color, so I allowed each coat to dry fully for around two minutes before adding the next.

I've used this gold hair mascara by Fekkai on many different eyebrows, and I find that it works best on thick, dark eyebrows. Three other great colored brow gels are Anastasia Beverly Hills Tinted Brow Gel, Kryolan Aquacolor Hair Mascara, and Medis Sun Glow Hair Mascara.

Often, though, if I don't have a specific color on hand, I will customize my own eyebrow gels by mixing clear brow gel with pigment. To avoid any clumps, I blend the gel and pigment on a mixing plate using a spatula, then use a clean mascara wand to apply the colored gel to the eyebrows.

Lace Up

For intricate makeup in a flash, these delicate vinyl cutouts developed by makeup artist Phyllis Cohen produce incredibly beautiful results.

BASE
MAC Pro Full Coverage Foundation in NC20.
Make Up For Ever HD Powder to set.

CONTOUR
MAC Powder Blush in Taupe.

BLUSH
Yaby Eye Shadow in pp062 Tamarind (from the Yaby World of Pearl Paint palette).

HIGHLIGHT
MAC Mineralize Skinfinish in Shimpagne. (This product has been discontinued; Charlotte Tilbury Bar of Gold or Chanel Poudre Signée de Chanel Illuminating Powder are good alternatives.)

EYES
Yaby Eye Shadows in pp062 Tamarind and pp026 Amber (from the Yaby World of Pearl Paint palette) blended softly on the eyelids, up into the creases, and underneath the eyes.
MAC Glitter in Gold on the eyelids and inner corners.
MAC 30 Lash single lashes in Medium and Long on the top lashes. Black mascara on the top and bottom lashes.

LIPS
MAC Lip Erase in Pale.
MAC Glitter in Gold on the Cupid's bow.

STICKERS
Face Lace in Mini Eyelace Swirlyqueue, Pied Peepers, and Swirlyqueue.

I love Face Lace by Phyllis Cohen. Her designs are so beautiful and versatile. I like to customize them by cutting and mixing and matching the designs, but if you need something specific, the Face Lace team will create bespoke designs and colors.

After finishing the makeup, I started placing all the Face Lace designs I had mapped out beforehand. I applied Face Lace in Mini Eyelace Swirlyqueue around the eye, then enhanced around the bottom lashes with Pied Peepers and Swirlyqueue. I used Swirlyqueue again on the jawline and included a lot of single smaller Face Lace stickers in my design. These single stickers used to be sold in a multipack, but I haven't seen them available on Face Lace's website recently.

The application instructions of the stickers are very easy to follow. However, I made some mistakes. I should have washed my hands before touching and placing the Face Lace as I had makeup residue on my fingers, which transferred onto the stickers. I also added more contour to the cheek after applying the stickers, which marked them. If you look carefully, you can see the offending stickers below the inner corners of the eyes and across the cheekbones. It was so tempting to have this fixed in postproduction, but I wanted to share this so readers can see the attention to detail required when shooting a beauty editorial.

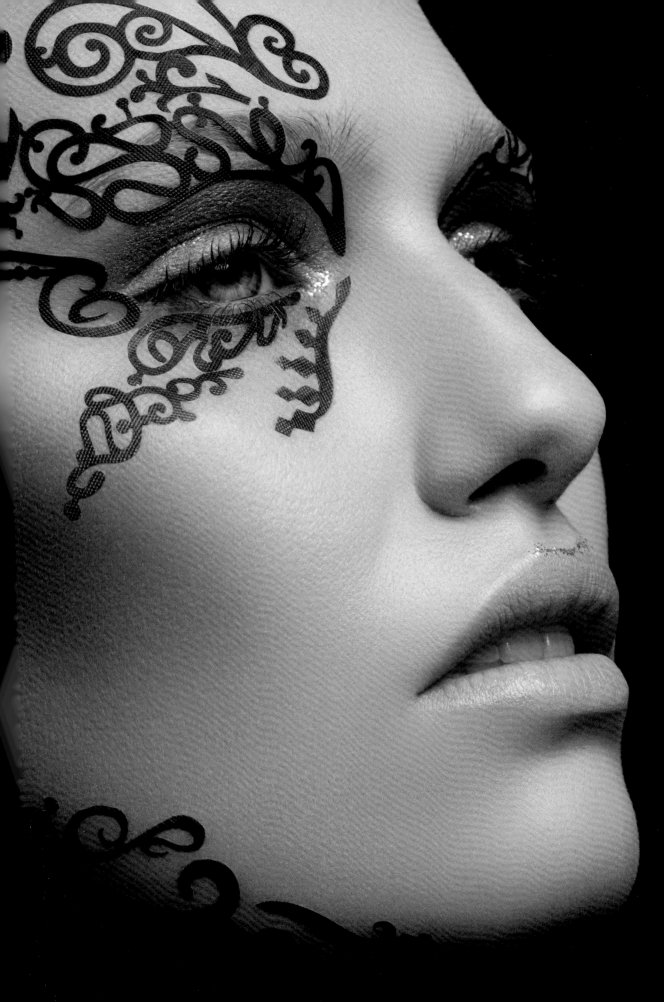

First Flush

Makeup artist Phylis Cohen's beautiful Face Lace stickers
leave mesmerizing patterns when used as a stencil. Just add blush.

BASE
MAC Pro Full Coverage
Foundation in NC15.
Make Up For Ever HD Powder
to set.

BLUSH
Kryolan blushes in R9 and Lake
(from the Kryolan Professional
Blusher Set 15 Colors).
Hakuhodo brushes 210 and 212
to apply.

CONTOUR
DiorSkin Poudre Shimmer
in 004 Diamond Pop.

EYES
Yaby Eye Shadows in pp05
Pink Tourmaline (from the
Yaby World of Pearl Paint
palette) on the eyelids
and underneath the eyes.
Becca Shimmering Skin
Perfector Pressed
Highlighter in Pearl on the
inner corners and on the
eyelids above the pupils.
MAC 30 Lash single lashes
in Medium and Long
on the top lashes.
Black mascara on the top
and bottom lashes.

LIPS
MAC Pro Full Coverage
Foundation in NC15 (whatever
is left on the brush).

STENCILS
Face Lace in Fleurty
around the eyes.
Face Lace Mehndoodle
Design 2 around the jawline.

As with the previous look, I used Phyllis Cohen's genius Face Lace again, but this time as a stencil. After finishing my foundation, I stuck Face Lace in Fleurty around the eyes. Sophia's eyebrows are so light that it worked perfectly; the beauty comes from seeing the whole stenciled effect uninterrupted by a strong eyebrow. If I had a model with dark, strong eyebrows, I would probably either glue the brows down with Elmer's All Purpose School Glue Stick (see Dream Weaver on page 76 for how to do this technique) and camouflage them, or design my look differently.

I used Face Lace Mehndoodle Design 2 around the jawline. It looked amazing, but I felt the lips weren't integrated with the rest of the face. To fix this issue, I cut off the two large flowers from the Face Lace Fleurty and added them on and around the lips.

To contour the stencil, I used Hakuhodo brushes 210 and 212 and applied a mixture of Kryolan blushes in R9 and Lake. To achieve these clean lines, I applied a lot of color, building it slowly and making sure I'd applied color below the jawline and slightly down the neck.

To finish, I added a little bit of DiorSkin Poudre Shimmer in 004 Diamond Pop to highlight the cheekbones, then carefully lifted the Face Lace stickers to reveal the final look. So beautiful!

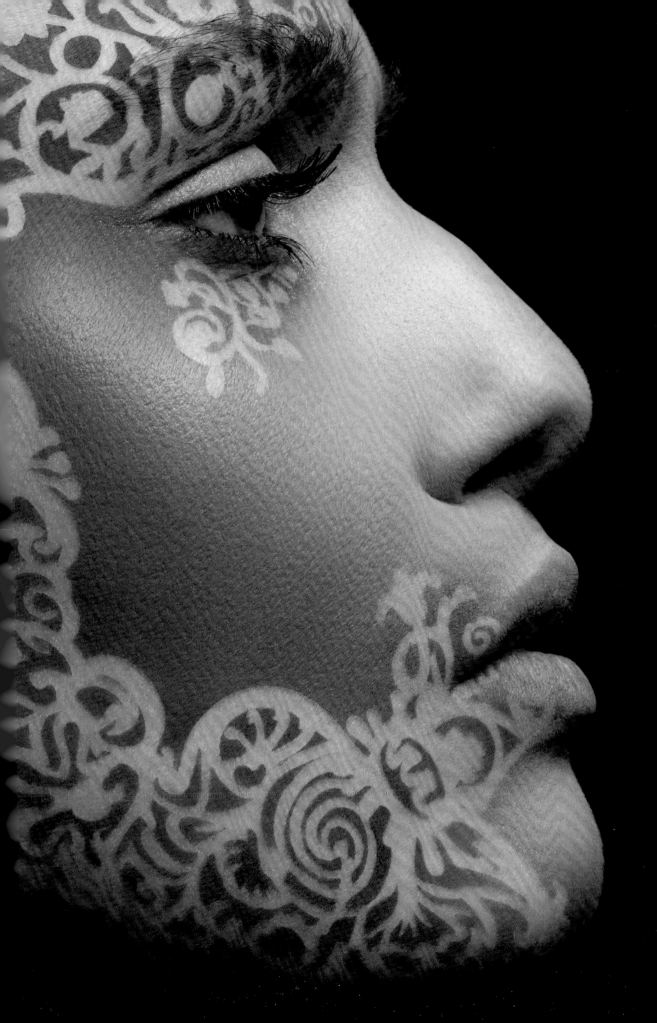

"It's worth spending time researching your model before a shoot. Look at her best and worst images to really understand the nuances of her face. This will help you create a look that is truly beautiful and unique, allowing the character of her face to shine."

Toni Malt

Gold Rush

This look takes inspiration from the beautiful gold-leafed eyes created by makeup artist Peter Philips for Fendi's Spring-Summer 2012 show. Makeup at its most precious.

BASE
Charlotte Tilbury Light Wonder Foundation in 4 Fair. Make Up For Ever HD Powder to set.

CONTOUR
Illamasqua Powder Blusher in Disobey.

BLUSH
Chanel Joues Contraste Powder Blush in 68 Rose Ecrin to warm and soften the skin tone on the cheeks.

EYES
MAC Fluidline in Blacktrack as eyeliner.
Eylure Girls Aloud Lashes in Nicola.
Black mascara on the top lashes only.
Illamasqua Pure Pigment in Breathe on the inner corners.
Kryolan Clear Glitter Gel applied with a MAC 239 Eye Shader Brush.
Imitation GoldLeaf Sheets.
Urban Decay Eye Shadow in Smog (from Urban Decay Naked eye shadow palette) to contour beneath the eyes with a MAC 219 Pencil Brush.

LIPS
Dior Addict Lipstick in 414 Sand.

I sourced these imitation gold-leaf sheets in the nail art section of a beauty supply store; they're featherlight and look just beautiful when applied to the skin.

I cut one gold sheet into tiny little pieces—it's worth being patient; thirty smaller pieces look so much nicer than three large pieces—then applied a thin layer of Kryolan Clear Glitter Gel over the eyes and eyebrows using a MAC 239 Eye Shader Brush. Using tweezers, I then gently placed the foil bits on top of the glue. It took me about forty-five minutes to place all the foil.

This look definitely needs the black eyeliner and black mascara—possibly even a pair of eyelashes. When I first created this look, I didn't use the black eyeliner and it looked awful, so I had to carefully work in the liner after I'd placed the foil. Take it from me, it's much easier to apply the liner before the foil!

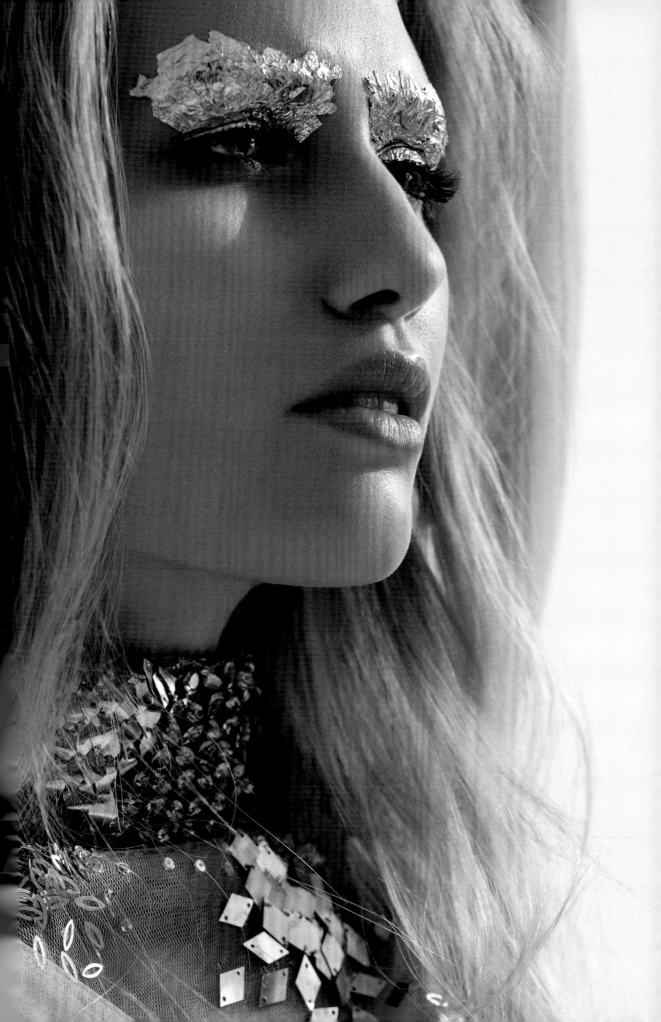

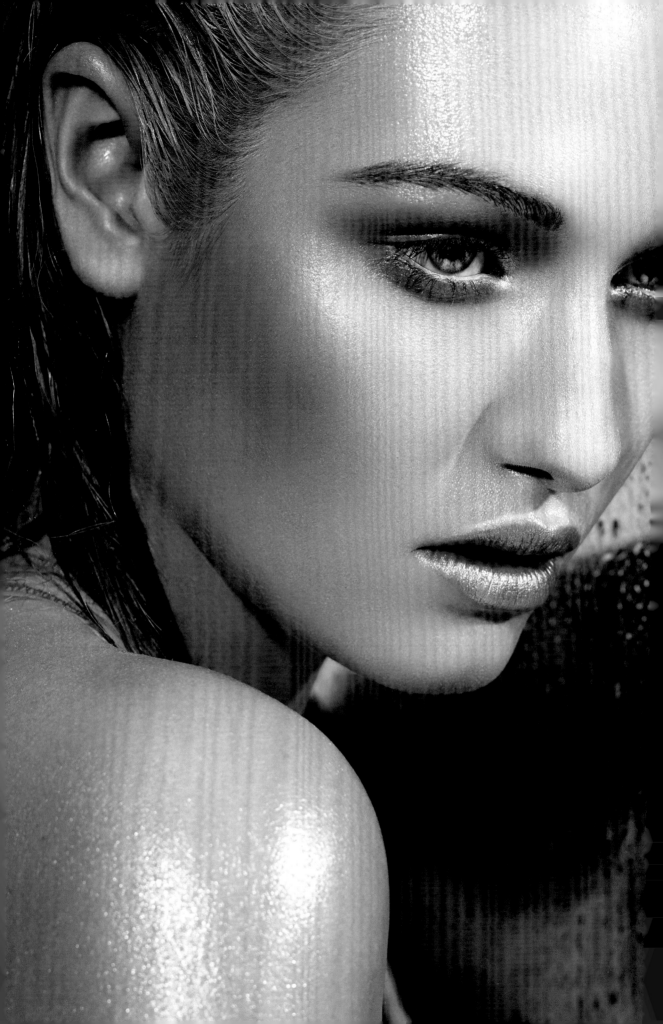

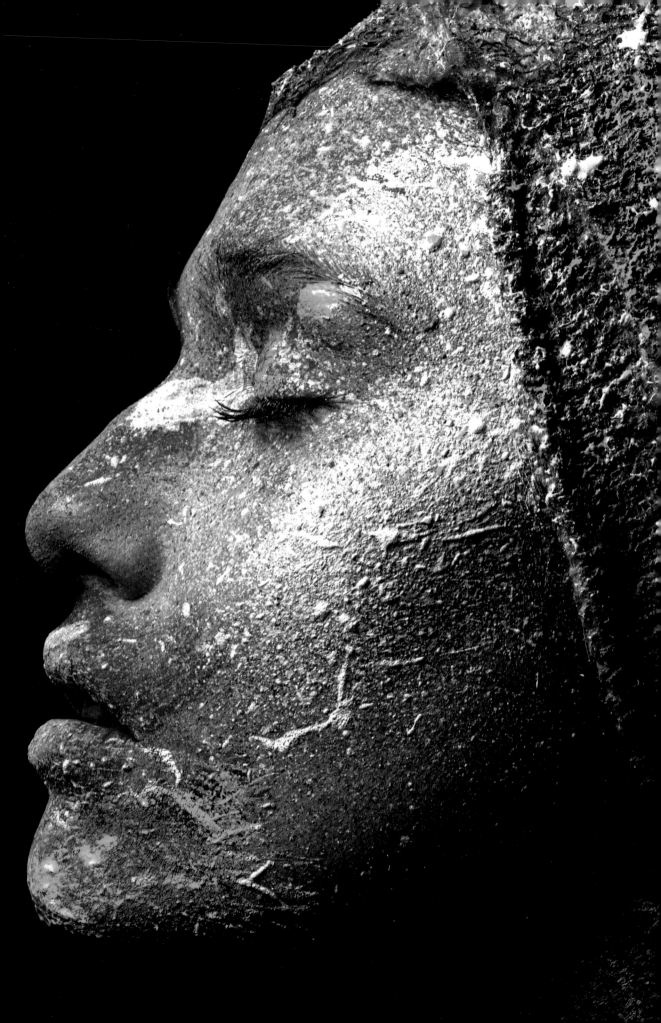

Light Fantastic

Decadent and magical, this look goes galactic with stunning crystal embellishment. Keep makeup softly blended and allow the light to do all the work.

BASE
Charlotte Tilbury Light Wonder Foundation in 4 Fair.

EYES
Urban Decay Eye Shadows in Smog and Dark Horse (from Urban Decay Naked eye shadow palette) to create a soft, very blended smoky eye.

Illamasqua Pure Pigment in Breath to set highlights on the inner corners. Lots of MAC 30 Lash single lashes in Long. Black mascara on the top and bottom lashes.

LIPS
MAC Pro Full Coverage Foundation in NC20 (just what's left on the brush) brushed over the lips. Vaseline to keep the lips moisturized.

CRYSTALS
Swarovski crystals. DUO eyelash adhesive.

I love embellishing the skin with Swarovski crystals because the finished look is so ethereal and decadent. This look is inspired by London-based makeup artist Lan Nguyen-Grealis. Lan's creations are out-of-this-world beautiful; she's definitely the queen of crystal face embellishment.

After finishing the makeup application, Sophia lay on the studio sofa so I could apply the crystals. She had just come back from New York the day before, so she was really tired; within minutes, she was fast asleep! From start to finish, this look took around two hours to create, so having Sophia asleep actually worked in my favor and gave me plenty of time.

When deciding where to place the crystals, I tend to stick to the makeup principles of highlighting. Never be afraid to experiment, though; breaking the rules can lead to the most unexpected, beautiful, and striking outcomes. Experiment with different sizes of crystals, too, as they reflect the light differently and give the finished look incredible depth.

DUO eyelash adhesive is ideal for applying crystals—just be aware that the larger, heavier crystals will need to pre-dry for five minutes before being placed on the skin.

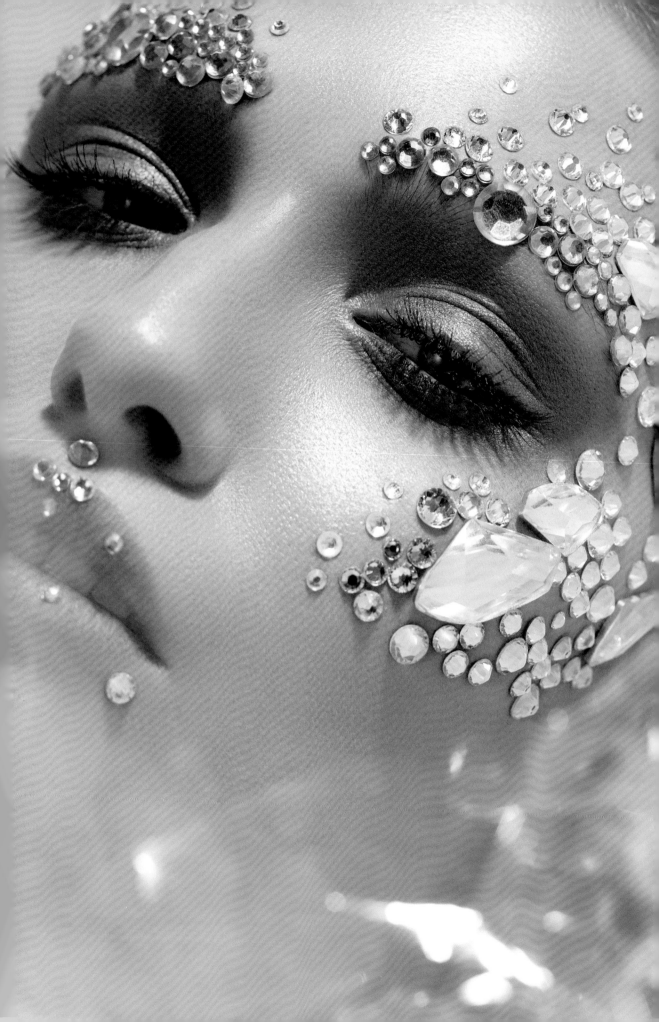

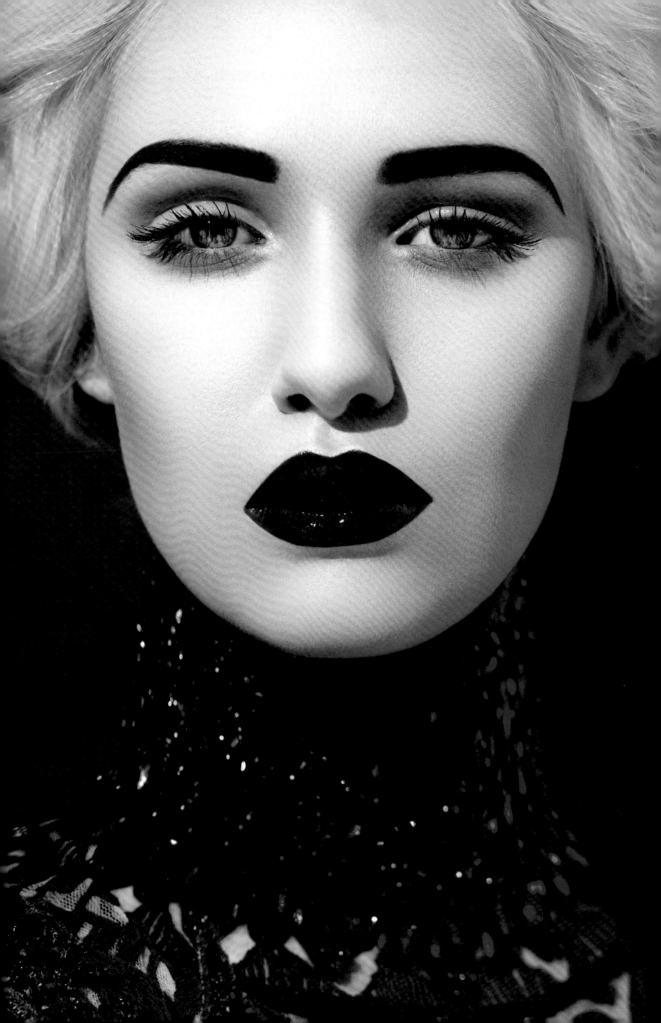

Scarlet Fever

THE FACE GETS A HIGH-DRAMA TRANSFORMATION AS BROWS AND LIPS ARE RAMPED RIGHT UP WITH A VIBRANT COLOR CHANGE.

BASE
MAC Pro Full Coverage Foundation in NC15. Make Up For Ever HD Powder to set.

HIGHLIGHT
Skin N Nature Cookie Marble Blusher in 01 Rose.

CONTOUR
MAC Powder Blush in Taupe.

EYES
MAC Powder Blush in Taupe to contour the eyes, above the creases, and lightly underneath the lower lashes. Illamasqua Pure Pigment in Breathe to highlight above the pupils and the inner corners. MAC 30 Lash single lashes in Medium and Long on the top lashes. MAC Clear Lipglass on the eyelids to add shine.

EYEBROWS
MAC Pro Pigment in Basic Red. MAC 231 Small Shader Brush to apply.

LIPS
Lip Pencil in Redd. Lancôme L'Absolu Rouge Lipstick in 132 Caprice. MAC Clear Lipglass applied generously.

EYEBROWS ARE SUCH A BEAUTIFUL ELEMENT TO PLAY WITH, AND THERE'S NO END TO WHAT YOU CAN DO WITH THEM. MAKEUP ARTIST PAT McGRATH'S SORBET-COLORED BROWS AT THE BALENCIAGA FALL-WINTER 2010 SHOW WERE SO BEAUTIFUL, AND THEY DEMONSTRATED HOW CHANGING EYEBROW COLOR CAN REALLY TRANSFORM A LOOK. HERE, I WANTED TO TRANSFORM THE BROWS INTO SOMETHING VERY DRAMATIC.

TO TURN THE BROWS A VIBRANT RED, I USED MAC PRO PIGMENT IN BASIC RED. I FIND MOST RED PIGMENTS ARE SLIGHTLY PINK, BUT THIS ONE BY MAC IS A FANTASTIC BLUE-RED. ANOTHER PRODUCT THAT WOULD WORK WELL FOR THIS LOOK IS YABY EYE SHADOW IN ES287 HIBISCUS FROM YABY'S SOMETHING BRIGHT PRE-SET EYE SHADOW PALETTE. I FIND THAT PIGMENT AND EYE SHADOWS REALLY GIVE A MORE STRIKING RESULT THAN CREAM COLORS.

RED STAINS THE SKIN AND IS A PAIN TO REMOVE, SO TAKE A LOT OF CARE WHEN APPLYING. TO AVOID COLOR FALLOUT, I MADE SURE I DIDN'T HAVE EXCESS PIGMENT ON MY BRUSH AND USED A SMALL MAC 23 BRUSH TO APPLY THE PIGMENT VERY CAREFULLY.

Shades of Gray

BLACK-AND-WHITE PHOTOGRAPHY REFINES
MAKEUP TO LIGHT AND DARK, SO KEEPING THINGS
SIMPLE AND MONOCHROMATIC IS KEY.
HERE, A LIPSTICK CHANGE HAS DRAMATIC IMPACT.

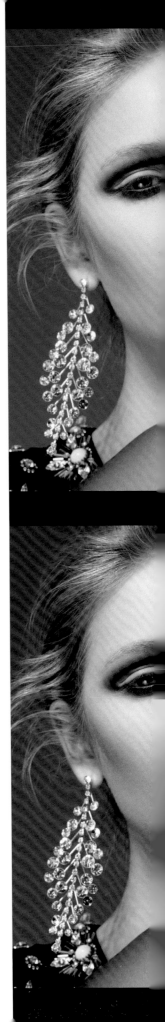

BASE
Charlotte Tilbury Light
Wonder Foundation in 2 Fair.

CONTOUR
Charlotte Tilbury Filmstar
Bronze & Glow.

EYES
Charlotte Tilbury Filmstar
Bronze & Glow (sculpting
color) to map out the shape,
gently blending outward

with a MAC 228 Mini Shader
Brush. Kevyn Aucoin
The Essential Eye Shadow
in N°110 Blackest Black to
define the shape and blend
areas further.
Illamasqua Pure Pigment
in Breathe to highlight
the inner corners.
MAC Eye Kohl in Fascinating
inside the waterlines.
One coat of black mascara
on the top and bottom lashes.

EYEBROWS
A small amount of MAC Pro
Full Coverage Foundation in
NC15 to lighten the eyebrows.
Disposable mascara wand.

LIPS
Vaseline.
Dolce & Gabbana Shine
Lipstick in 136 Love.
Illamasqua lipstick in Disciple.

I AM ALWAYS EXCITED WHEN I'M TOLD THAT AN EDITORIAL SHOOT WILL INCLUDE BLACK-AND-WHITE IMAGES. THERE IS SOMETHING SO SERENE ABOUT THESE PHOTOS. THE MONOCHROME BLACK DESIGN ON THE EYE AND THE BEAUTIFUL SCULPTED CHEEKS AND EXPERIMENTATION WITH THE LIPS SIMPLIFY BEAUTY TO FORM AND TEXTURE, LIGHT AND DARK.

I WANTED TO DEMONSTRATE HOW SOMETHING AS SIMPLE AS PICKING OUT A LIP COLOR CAN DRAMATICALLY CHANGE A BLACK-AND-WHITE IMAGE. FIRST, I SIMPLY ADDED VASELINE ON THE LIPS, AND THE LOOK IS YOUNG, FRESH, AND MODERN—THE SORT OF MAKEUP THAT WOULD SUIT AN EDITORIAL SHOOT. THE PINK LIPSTICK MADE IT FAR MORE SOPHISTICATED—SOMETHING I'D CONSIDER FOR A JEWELRY CAMPAIGN. THE DEEP NAVY LIPSTICK LOOKED ALMOST BLACK IN THE BLACK-AND-WHITE IMAGE AND INSTANTLY GAVE A RETRO FEEL. TO GET A PERFECT FINISH WHEN WORKING IN BLACK AND WHITE, THINK ABOUT PRODUCTS AS SHADES OF GRAY AND WORK OUT HOW THEY WILL TRANSLATE IN THE FINAL IMAGE. BLUSHES, FOR EXAMPLE, TEND TO LOOK DIRTY IN BLACK AND WHITE, SO I SKIP THEM. IT'S BETTER TO KEEP THINGS SIMPLE BY FOCUSING ON CONTOUR AND HIGHLIGHT.

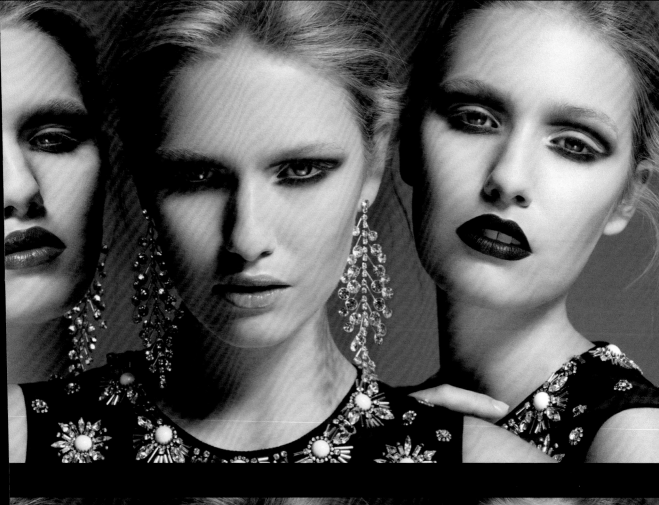

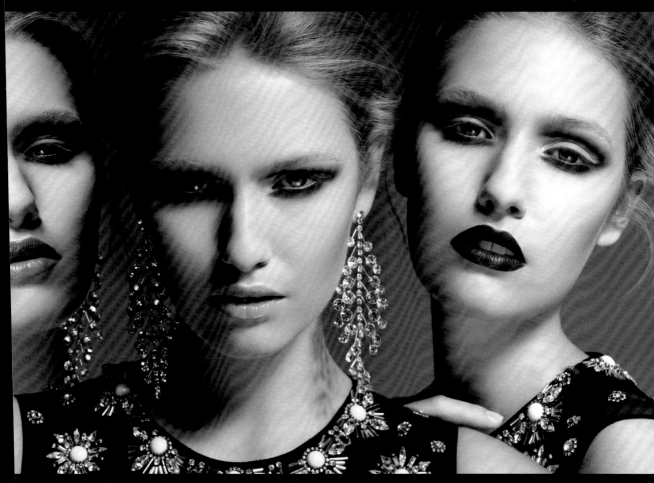

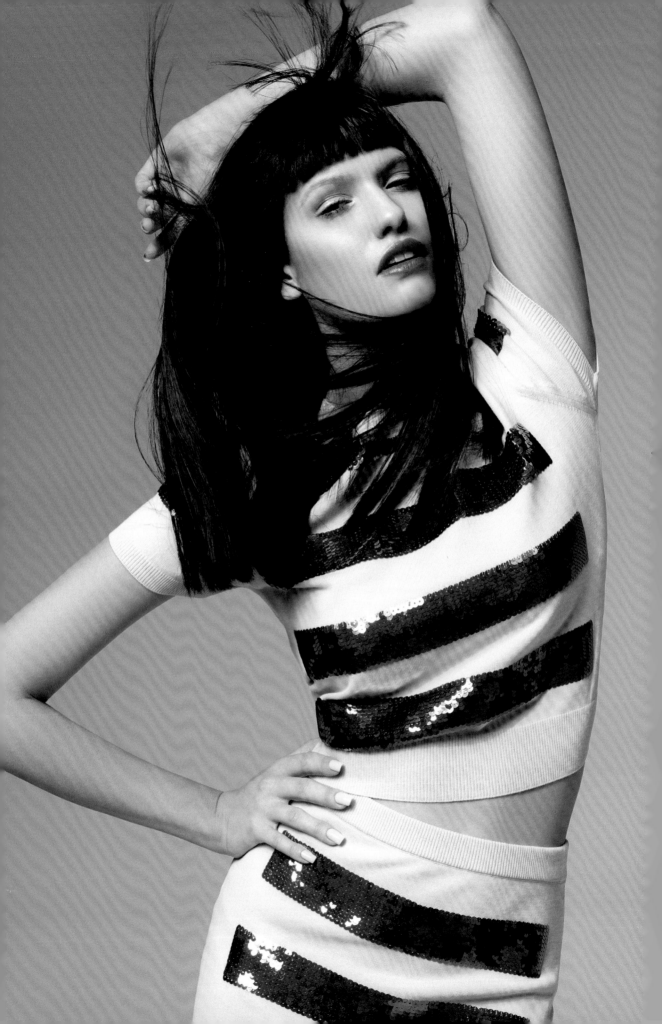

Pop To It

With vibrant hues and standout prints taking center stage, makeup takes on a supporting role. Here, the look is clean and pretty with a shot of punchy pink.

BASE
Charlotte Tilbury Light Wonder Foundation in 2 Fair. Make Up For Ever HD Powder to set.

HIGHLIGHT
Skin N Nature Cookie Marble Blusher in 01 Rose.

CONTOUR
MAC Powder Blush in Taupe.

EYES
MAC Matte Eye Shadow in Wedge to contour very softly in the creases and underneath the eyes. Illamasqua Pure Pigment in Breathe on the inner corners and all over the eyelids. MAC Eye Kohl in Fascinating on the waterlines. Black mascara.

EYEBROWS
A small amount of MAC Pro Full Coverage Foundation in NC15 brushed through the eyebrows to lighten. Disposable mascara wand.

LIPS
MAC Lip Pencil in Embrace Me to outline and fill the lips. MAC Lipstick in Show Orchid. MAC Clear Lipglass.

There was so much going on with the hair and clothes in this pop art–inspired look that I thought the best option was to play down the makeup and allow the fashion and hair to shine. I also knew that we were going to add illustrations to the images, so I wanted the makeup to be subtle. This makeup relies entirely on shading and highlighting the face and eyes, with a punch of color on the lips to finish.

Whenever I receive a brief, I have to keep in mind whether it's for fashion editorial or beauty editorial, because the makeup can be very different. I wanted to use this fashion shoot to highlight how sometimes, even if a brief sounds really exciting, with endless makeup opportunities, it's better to take a step back—which can be hard!

I've kept this makeup very clean and simple so that the clothes can take center stage, but if I had received the same brief for a beauty shoot, I would have done completely different makeup, creating a much more outspoken, playful, and vibrant feel.

Loud Mouth

Violent Lips temporary tattoos add instant fierceness and fullness. No wonder they're such a smash hit with songstresses such as Lady Gaga, Katy Perry, and Jessie J.

BASE
MAC Pro Full Coverage Foundation in NC20. Make Up For Ever HD Powder to set.

LIPS
Violent Lips Temporary Lip Appliqués in Coral Giraffe. Scissors, cotton balls, and water to prepare the lip tattoo.

There are so many fun makeup products hitting the shelves right now, and Violent Lips Temporary Lip Appliqués are a great one to try.

Here, I used Coral Giraffe because the pattern is strong and bold while still being pretty. Starting with clean, product-free lips, I popped the appliqué out of its stencil and measured it against Sophia's lips. I love a rounded, full top lip, so I cut the transfer into a beautiful rounded shape before peeling the plastic film off the appliqué. I then asked Sophia to keep her lips wide open while I put the sticky side of the tattoo on her lips. Next I used a cotton ball soaked in water to wet the backing paper until it started to come off. Once the paper was gone, I smoothed the tattoo with a cotton swab, again soaked in water. The temporary tattoo took about five minutes to fully dry.

Much to my surprise, the tattoo looked flawless when the lips were closed. However, in the images where Sophia's lips are parted, it was easy to see where the tattoos end at the inner corners of the lips. Despite many attempts to fix this issue on the shoot day, we needed to fix these demarcation lines in postproduction by blending the tattoo into the inner corners of the lip. The other issue I had with these tattoos is that they have a slight sheen to them. I prefer a matte finish, which is also something we had to achieve in postproduction.

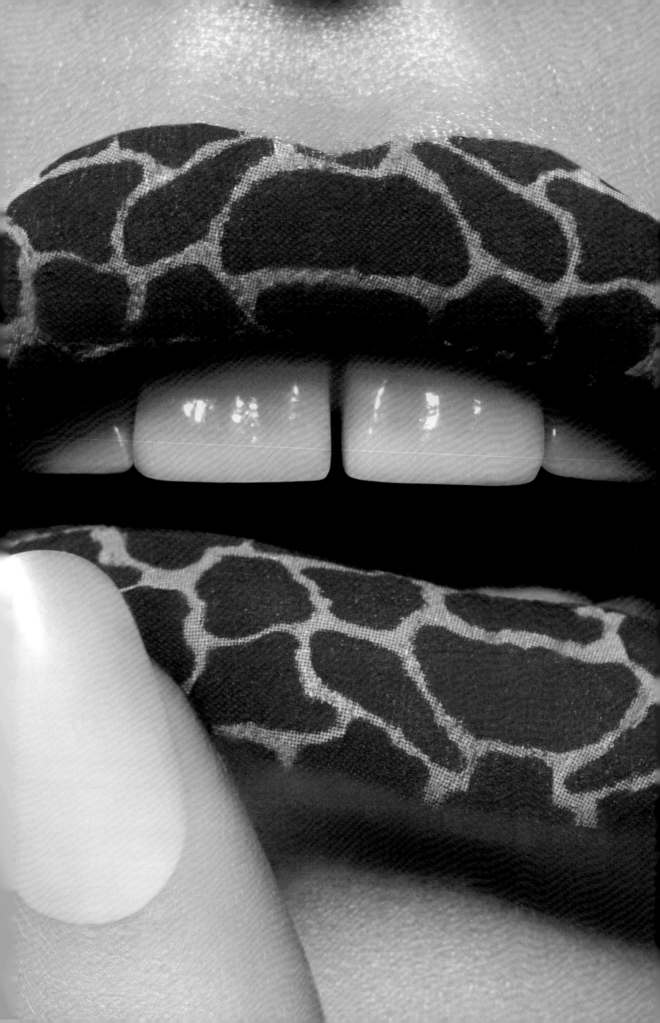

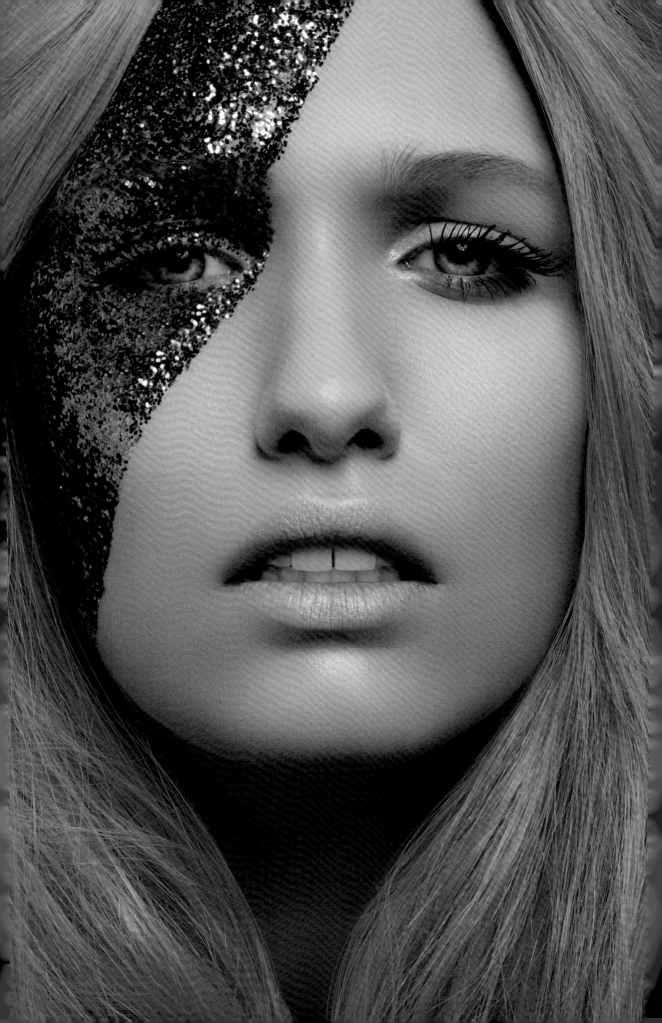

Boogie Nights

GLITTER SHAPES GIVE MAKEUP INSTANT STAR-STUDDED APPEAL.
INSPIRED BY DAVID BOWIE'S *ALADDIN SANE* ALBUM COVER,
THIS GLITTERING BLUE SLASH IS PURE GLAM ROCK.

BASE
MAC Pro Full Coverage
Foundations in NC20
and NC30 (mixed).
Make Up For Ever HD
Powder to set.

CONTOUR
MAC Powder Blush in Taupe.

EYES
MAC Powder Blush in Taupe to
lightly contour the creases and
underneath the lower lashes.
Illamasqua Pure Pigment in
Breathe on the inner corners.
MAC Eye Kohl in Fascinating
on the waterlines.
MAC 3 Lash single lashes
in Medium and Long
applied to the top lashes.
Black mascara.

EYEBROWS
Brushed up and outward.

LIPS
MAC Lip Erase in Pale mixed
with a small amount of Make Up
For Ever Flash Color in 02 Coral.

GLITTER
Make Up For Ever Pro Only
Medium Size Glitters in N51
Blue Peacock.
Make Up For Ever Mist & Fix.
Bobbi Brown Eye Sweep brush.

GLITTER HAS SUCH AN IMPACT WHEN PHOTOGRAPHED, AND THIS IS A FANTASTIC TECHNIQUE TO MASTER BECAUSE IT ALLOWS YOU TO CREATE ALMOST ANY GLITTER SHAPE ON THE FACE.

AFTER I FINISHED ALL THE MAKEUP, I APPLIED TWO STRIPS OF SURGICAL TAPE ACROSS SOPHIA'S FACE TO MARK WHERE I WANTED THE GLITTER TO GO. I THEN SPRAYED MAKE UP FOR EVER MIST & FIX BETWEEN THE TWO STRIPS OF TAPE, KEEPING THE SPRAY BOTTLE ABOUT FOUR INCHES AWAY FROM THE FACE. AFTER LETTING THE MAKEUP FIXER DRY FOR ABOUT THIRTY SECONDS, I GENTLY PRESSED THE GLITTER INTO THE WET AREA USING A BOBBI BROWN EYE SWEEP BRUSH.

TO ACHIEVE THIS FULL-COVERAGE EFFECT, IT'S IMPORTANT TO TAKE YOUR TIME AND USE DOUBLE THE AMOUNT OF GLITTER YOU THINK YOU NEED. I REMOVED THE TAPE BY PEELING SLOWLY UPWARD FROM THE BASE, THEN CLEANED AWAY ANY GLITTER FALLOUT BY PRESSING AND LIFTING A SMALL PIECE OF SURGICAL TAPE ON THE GLITTER SPOTS. I FINISHED THE LOOK BY CLEANING UP ANY AREAS OF FOUNDATION THAT HAD BEEN DAMAGED BY THE TAPE.

IF YOU DON'T WANT THE DENT ABOVE THE EYEBROW, YOU CAN USE TWO PIECES OF TAPE TO STRAIGHTEN OUT THE LINE. I LIKED THE DENT AND WANTED TO KEEP IT BECAUSE IT REMINDED ME A LITTLE OF THE FAMOUS DAVID BOWIE *ALADDIN SANE* ALBUM COVER.

"Trick the mind into thinking there is no foundation on the skin by adding a hint of MAC Penultimate Brow Marker onto the tiniest of beauty spots after finishing the complexion. If the eye can see them, the mind believes it is bare skin."

Toni Malt

The New Matte

Forget cakey dullness—modern matte makeup is velvety smooth and softly focused. Get the look right and it's equally as vibrant and fresh as a dewy finish.

BASE
MAC Pro Full Coverage Foundation in NC20. Make Up For Ever HD Powder to set.

CONTOUR
Charlotte Tilbury Filmstar Bronze & Glow.

HIGHLIGHT
MAC Pro Full Coverage Foundation in NC15.

EYES
Chanel Écriture de Chanel Eyeliner Pen in 10 Noir. MAC 33 Lash false lash bundles. Bobbi Brown Eye Shadows in 18 Sable, 6 Gray, and 16 Slate. Illamasqua Liquid Metal in Enrapture.

EYEBROWS
Inglot Brow Powders in 569 and 560.

LIPS
Obsessive Compulsive Cosmetics Lip Tar in Uber. Make Up For Ever HD Powder to set.

Like most makeup artists, I have spent years perfecting my highlighting skills; I'm always in search of the perfect products to add that subtle illumination to skin. In recent years, going all matte seems almost forbidden. But an all-matte look can be so beautiful—rather than being dry and cakey, the new matte is velvety and full of life.

To achieve a velvet finish without dullness, I use a semi-matte or matte foundation. For this look, I applied MAC Pro Full Coverage Foundation, then set the skin with the amazing HD transparent powder from Make Up For Ever to keep it looking vibrant rather than cakey.

Bobbi Brown matte brown eye shadows are a mainstay in my kit. They are highly pigmented and photograph beautifully. Here, I mixed Sable, Gray, and Slate to create a large smoky eye that extended all the way up to the eyebrows. Of course, I couldn't help myself and decided to add a tiny highlight in the inner corners of the eyes using Illamasqua Liquid Metal in Enrapture. I felt it helped tie the eyes in with the beautiful rusty bronze colors of the background.

For the lip, I used OCC Lip Tar in Uber. I then patted the color down with a tissue and mattified with Make Up For Ever HD Powder.

I am definitely one of those makeup artists who love shine and dewiness, so I am almost surprised at how much I adore this velvet matte look. I'll absolutely be creating more matte skin in the future!

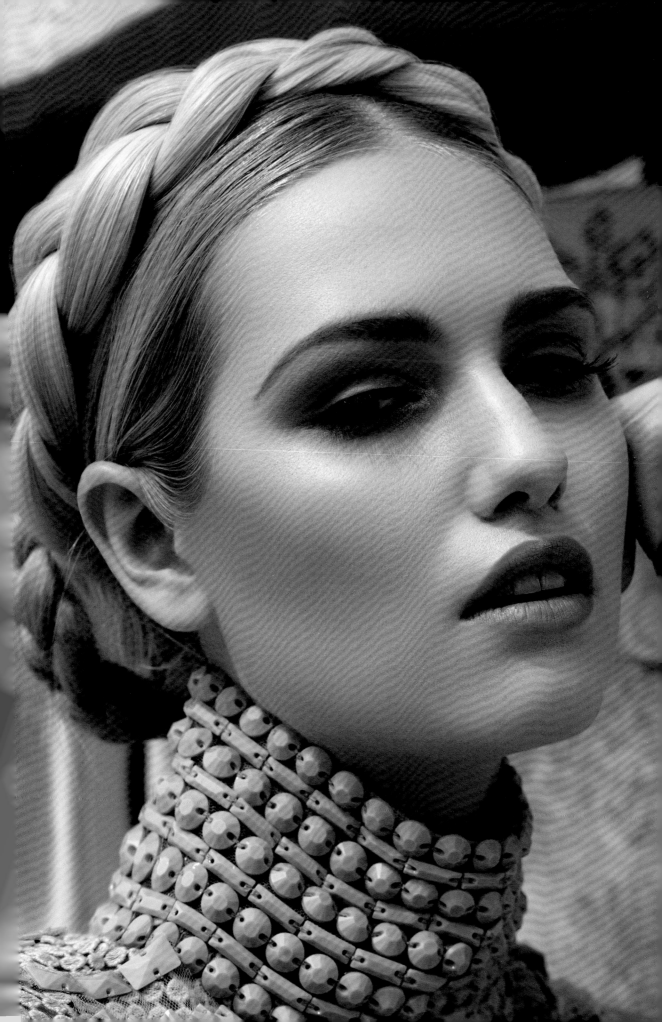

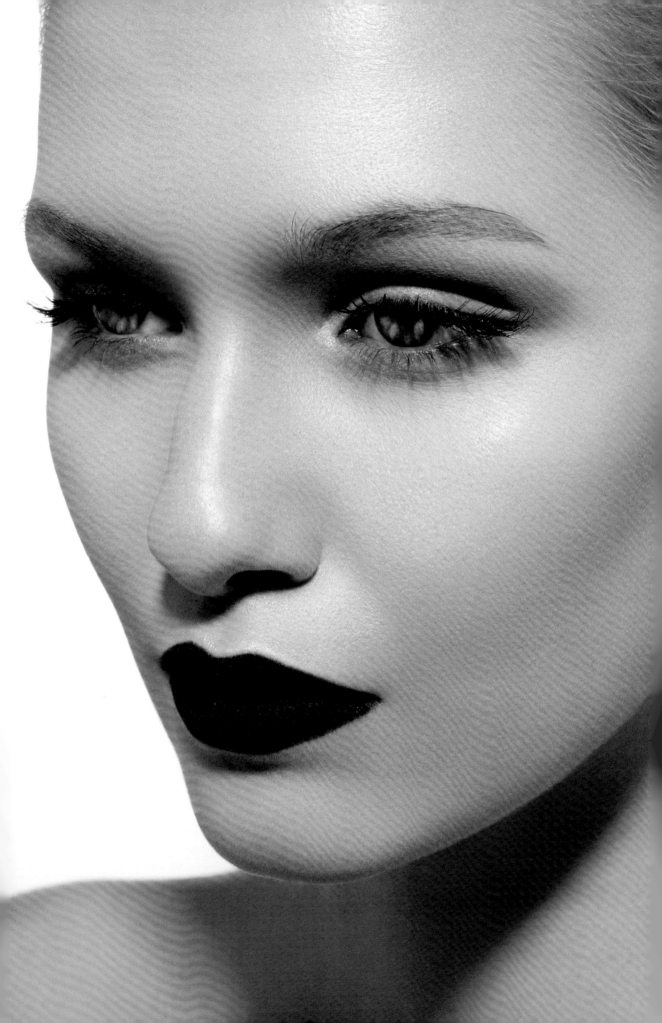

Simply Red

Some of the most intriguing looks come from experimenting with products. Lips get lacquered with a velvet topcoat for a look that's as seductive as a pair of plush red heels.

BASE
MAC Pro Full Coverage
Foundations in NC15
and NC20 (mixed).
Make Up For Ever HD Powder
to set around the nose,
middle of the forehead,
and under the eyes.

HIGHLIGHT
Skin N Nature Cookie Marble
Blusher in 01 Rose.

EYES
MAC Eye Shadow in Brun over
the eyelids and a little bit
more in the creases applied
with a large eye shadow
blending brush.
Becca Shimmering Skin
Perfector Pressed Highlighter
in Pearl on the inner corners.
MAC 3 Lash single lashes
in Medium and Long
on the top lashes.
One coat of black mascara.

LIPS
MAC Lip Pencil in Redd.
Lancôme L'Absolu Rouge
Lipstick in 132 Caprice.
Ciaté Wow Kit in Red Velvet.
MAC 231 Small Shader Brush.

Ciaté Wow Kits have been a big hit on the runway and in editorials. These manicure kits can create all sorts of amazing three-dimensional effects, such as caviar, metallic, glow-in-the-dark neon, and velvet.

For this look, I used the velvet topcoat on the lips. I had never used this technique on lips before, so I was excited to see how it would look when photographed. To be honest, I was not prepared for how amazingly this turned out. The result was stunning—so three-dimensional with beautiful gradations from light to dark.

To create the lip, I first applied a base using MAC Lip Pencil in Redd, followed by my favorite fire engine-red Lancôme L'Absolu Rouge Lipstick in 132 Caprice. I then gently pressed the Ciaté Red Velvet onto the lip using a MAC 231 brush. This takes time, as you need to be precise—and more is definitely more here.

When you think you are finished, pile on the same amount of Red Velvet again to achieve this full-coverage, multifaceted red. It took me about thirty minutes to prepare the lip.

I wanted to make sure the lips had maximum impact, so I kept the rest of the makeup to a minimum and allowed the lips to take center stage. I can't wait for the opportunity to do this again!

A Winter's Tale

This whimsical winter look is inspired by Peter Philips, currently Dior's creative and image director and previously Chanel's global creative director, who broke all the rules with his printed eyelids at Chanel's Fall-Winter 2010 show. This is sophistication at its purest.

BASE
Chanel Perfection Lumière in 12 Beige Rose.
Chanel Poudre Universelle Libre Natural Finish Loose Powder in 30 Naturel to set.

CONTOUR
Illamasqua Blusher in Disobey.

HIGHLIGHT
Skin N Nature Cookie Marble Blusher in 01 Rose.

BLUSH
Chanel Joues Contraste in 60 Rose Temptation.

EYES
Chanel Les 4 Ombres Quadra Eye Shadow in Prelude (darkest shade) to create a wash of color on the eyelids.
MAC Eye Kohl in Fascinating on the waterlines.
Black mascara on the top and bottom lashes.

EYEBROWS
Left natural.

LIPS
MAC Lip Pencil in Subculture.
Dior Addict Lip Maximizer to create a soft pink nude color.

I get so excited about new makeup techniques, and I just love breaking the rules of makeup to create something unique—so when I saw Peter Philips's stunning wintery eyes at the Chanel Ready-to-Wear Fall-Winter 2010 show, where he re-created in makeup the print Karl Lagerfeld used for his handbags and shoes, I knew I had to try it.

To create the eyes, I added <u>heaps of black mascara</u> onto a clean mascara wand and, using the same principle as for a smoky eye, pressed it into the creases before gently moving the wand in random outward strokes toward the eyebrows. I also added a few strokes underneath the lower lashes. To maintain the graphic <u>look</u> of these eyes, I made sure it was possible to see the strokes of the mascara bristles on the skin.

I was really excited by the results, but I have to laugh, because although this image looks wintery, we actually shot it outside the studio in Dubai's scorching 108°F heat. Sophia was standing under the only European-looking tree we could find among all those beautiful palms.

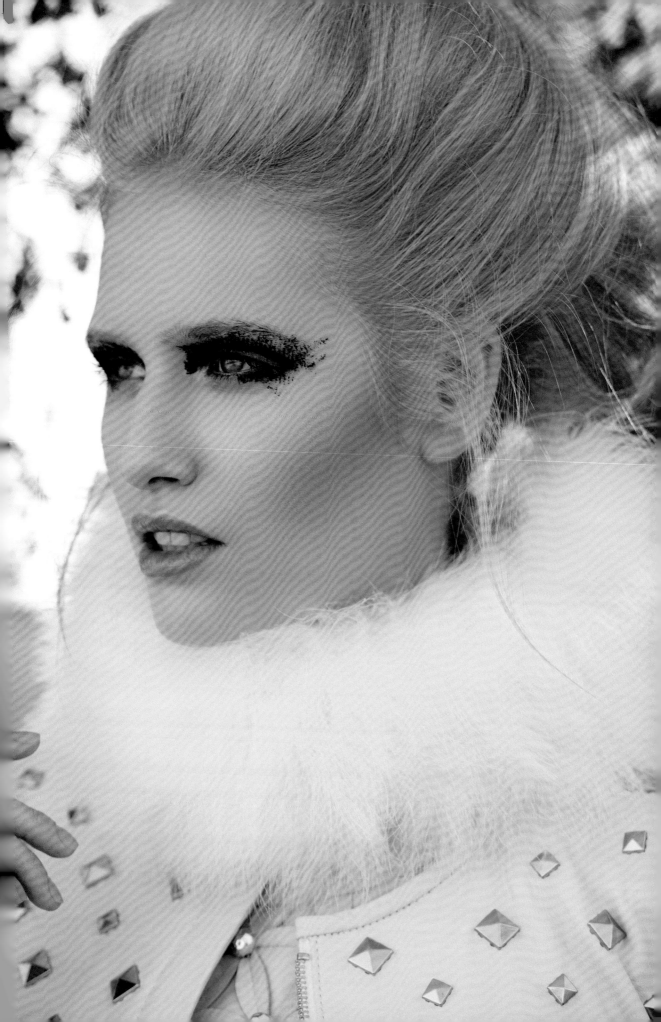

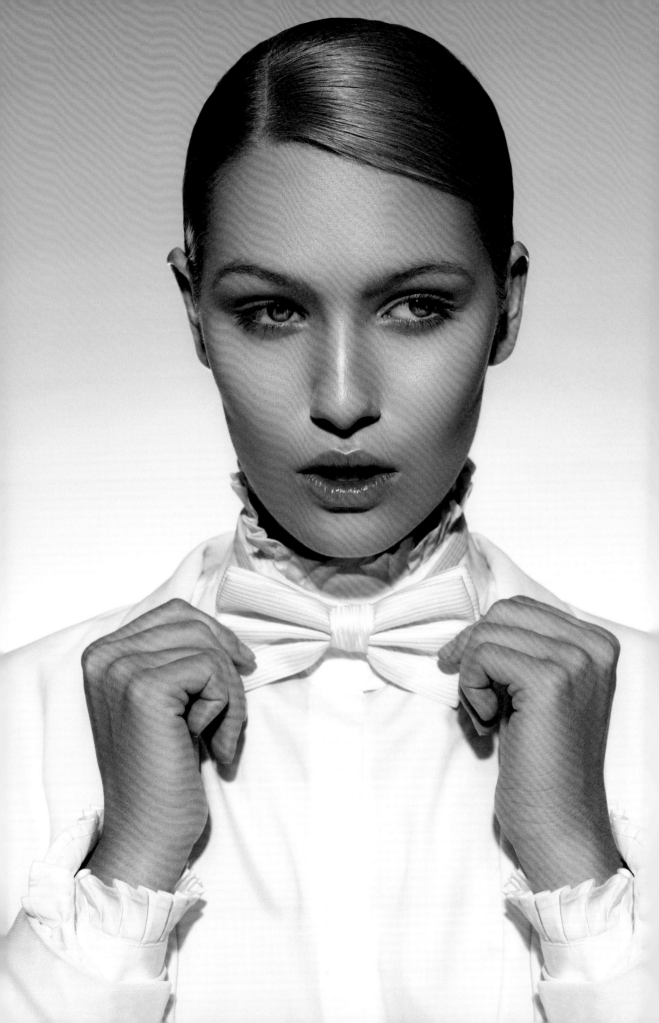

About a Boy

ANDROGYNY IS A LOOK OFTEN REQUESTED BY FASHION EDITORS. THE KEY TO GETTING IT RIGHT: GOOD SKIN PREPARATION, LIGHT-TOUCH FOUNDATION, AND BARELY-THERE CONTOURING.

SKIN PREP
Charlotte Tilbury's Multi-Miracle Glow cleanser, mask, and balm.
Charlotte Tilbury
Charlotte's Magic Cream.

BASE
Charlotte Tilbury Light Wonder Foundations in 2 and 4 Fair.
No setting powder was used for this look.

CONTOUR
MAC Powder Blush in Taupe.

EYES
MAC Matte Eye Shadow in Wedge to softly contour the creases and add depth underneath the lower lashes.
Illamasqua Pure Pigment in Breathe applied on the inner corners.
MAC Eye Kohl in Fascinating on the waterlines.
Dark brown mascara to enhance the eyelashes.

EYEBROWS
Ever-so-slightly enhanced using MAC Eye Brows pencil in Lingering and Fling.
Soften strokes by running a clean mascara wand through the brows multiple times.

LIPS
A little Vaseline applied with the finger.
A little Illamasqua Pure Pigment in Breathe on the Cupid's bow.

THIS LOOK RELIES STRONGLY ON GREAT SKIN PREPARATION, USING AS LITTLE FOUNDATION AS POSSIBLE AND SHADING EVER SO SOFTLY. TO PREP THE SKIN, I USED CHARLOTTE TILBURY'S MULTI-MIRACLE GLOW MASK, WHICH I LEFT ON FOR ABOUT TEN MINUTES, WASHED OFF WITH WATER, THEN FOLLOWED WITH CHARLOTTE TILBURY CHARLOTTE'S MAGIC CREAM. I CAN'T LIVE WITHOUT THESE TWO PRODUCTS, ESPECIALLY WHEN SHOOTING BEAUTY EDITORIALS WHERE YOUR MODEL'S SKIN NEEDS TO STAY IN PERFECT SHAPE ALL DAY.

THE KEY TO THIS LOOK IS IN THE SHADING. INSTEAD OF CREATING RAZOR-SHARP CHEEKBONES, I CREATED A MUCH MORE MASCULINE FEEL BY PLACING SOFT CONTOURS BELOW THE CHEEKBONES AND PULLING THE COLOR RIGHT DOWN TOWARD EITHER SIDE OF THE MOUTH. IT'S IMPORTANT TO KEEP THE CONTOUR COLOR NEUTRAL AND STAY AWAY FROM ORANGE TONES. HERE, I USED MAC POWDER BLUSH IN TAUPE, BUT I ALSO COULD HAVE CHOSEN ILLAMASQUA POWDER BLUSHER IN DISOBEY—BOTH ARE PERFECT FOR THIS LOOK.

SOPHIA HAS REALLY LIGHT HAIR AND BROWS, SO I DIDN'T FEEL THAT MAKING HER EYEBROWS STRONGER WOULD HAVE BEEN THE RIGHT WAY TO GO TO ACHIEVE AN ANDROGYNOUS LOOK. IF, HOWEVER, I HAD BEEN WORKING WITH A DARK-HAIRED MODEL, I WOULD HAVE CONSIDERED MAKING THE EYEBROWS MUCH STRONGER IN A MANLY KIND OF WAY.

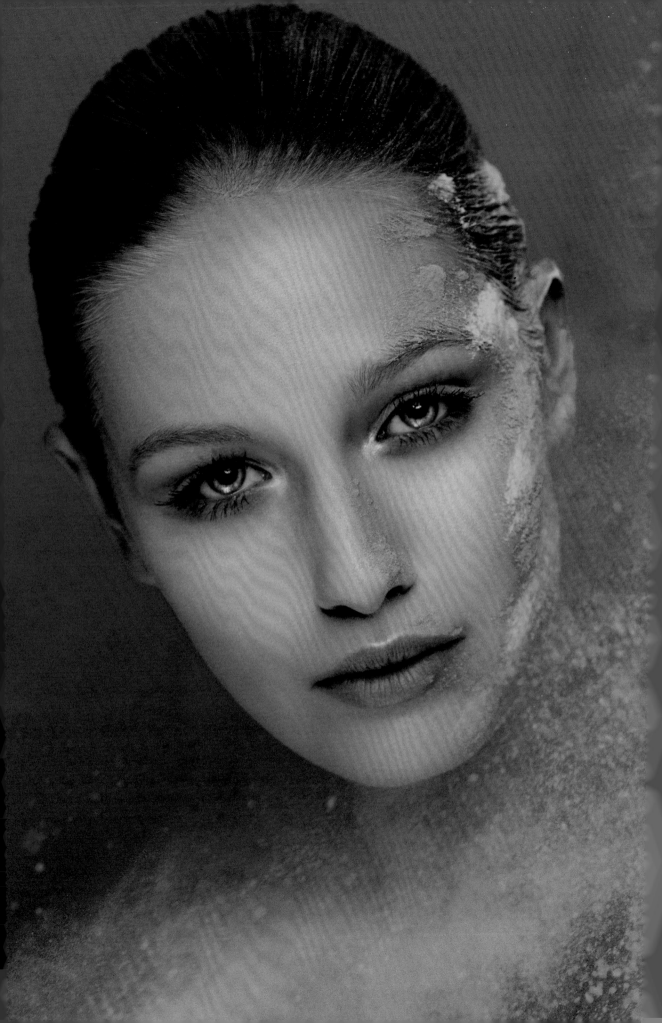

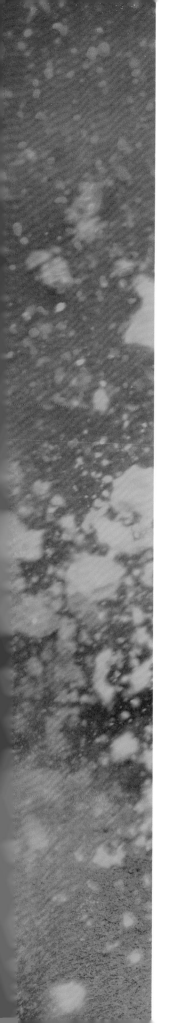

Color Blast

Standout blue eyes are easily achieved with MAC Pro Paint Sticks in your arsenal. Take the color way up to the brows and pile on the lashes.

BASE
Charlotte Tilbury Light Wonder Foundation in 2 Fair. Make Up For Ever HD Powder to set.

CONTOUR
MAC Mineralize Skinfinish Natural in Medium Dark.

EYES
MAC Pro Paint Stick in Hi-Def Cyan applied with a MAC 217 Blending Brush all over the lids up to the eyebrows and underneath the eyes. MAC Pro Paint Stick in Marine Ultra to enhance the creases. MAC Chromagraphic Pencil in Marine Ultra on the waterlines. Illamasqua Pure Pigment in Breathe in the inner corners. MAC 30 Lash single lashes in Short applied to the bottom lash lines. MAC 30 Lash in Medium applied to the top lash lines. Six coats of MAC Zoom Lash in Blue Charge applied over the lashes.

EYEBROWS
Eyebrows were left natural: simply brushed up and outward.

LIPS
Rimmel Lasting Finish Lipstick by Kate Moss in 26.

This is a really quick way to add powerful color to the eyes. I applied MAC Pro Paint Sticks (one of my favorite products) to the eyelids, taking the color right up to the eyebrows. I also added color below the lower lash lines to add to the drama. I then set the blue with Make Up For Ever HD Powder for a look that was bold, beautiful, and matte.

MAC Pro Paint Sticks are so highly pigmented that I'm able to achieve full color payoff using very little product, which helps minimize creasing on the eyelids. Some lesser-quality eye shadows can lose their vibrancy under the photographer's lighting, but this will never happen with MAC Pro Paint Sticks. In terms of lighting, your eye makeup will look exactly the way you intend it to on camera. Because this product can look either wet or matte, I also use it as a base to add extra intensity to metallic eye shadows.

Surrealist Blue

MEXICAN PAINTER FRIDA KAHLO CONTINUES TO INSPIRE. HERE, THE MAKEUP ARTIST BECOMES THE PAINTER, AND THE MODEL HER CANVAS. RULES ARE DEFIANTLY BROKEN FOR A LOOK THAT'S SURREAL YET MESMERIZINGLY BEAUTIFUL.

BASE
MAC Pro Full Coverage Foundation in W10.
Lots of Make Up For Ever HD Powder to set.

HIGHLIGHT
MAC Pro Paint Sticks in Hi-Def Cyan and Pure White (mixed).

BLUSH
MAC Pro Paint Sticks in Genuine Orange and Process Magenta (mixed). Illamasqua Blusher Brush.

EYES
MAC Pro Paint Sticks in True Chartreuse applied with a MAC 217 Blending Brush. Charlotte Tilbury The Feline Flick in Panther as eyeliner. Black mascara on the top and bottom lashes.

EYEBROWS
MAC Eye Brows pencils in Lingering and Stud mixed and applied in small, upward strokes for a realistic finish.

LIPS
MAC Lipstick in Morange. Make Up For Ever HD Powder dabbed on top with a MAC 239 Eye Shader Brush to mattify the lipstick and give it full coverage.

MEXICAN PAINTER FRIDA KAHLO IS A PERSONA I HAVE BEEN ASKED TO REINTERPRET MANY TIMES BY FASHION EDITORS. SHE WAS A WONDERFULLY UNIQUE SURREALIST PAINTER AND, IN MY MIND, ONE OF THE MOST REVOLUTIONARY AND INFLUENTIAL WOMAN IN MODERN CULTURE— PARTICULARLY FROM A MAKEUP AND HAIR POINT OF VIEW.

FRIDA'S LOOK IS DEFINED BY HER UNIBROW AND BRAIDED FLOWER HAIR, SO THOSE ELEMENTS ARE PORTRAYED IN THIS LOOK. HOWEVER, I ALSO WANTED TO CAPTURE THE FACT THAT FRIDA WAS, OF COURSE, A PAINTER. THROUGH MY MAKEUP, I WANTED TO USE SOPHIA'S FACE AS THE CANVAS FOR A PAINTING. I USED MAC PRO PAINT STICKS FOR THE ENTIRE LOOK BECAUSE IT GAVE ME SO MUCH COLOR FLEXIBILITY AND ALLOWED ME TO BLEND AND CUSTOMIZE EACH HUE. FOR THE HIGHLIGHTS ON THE CHEEKS, I MIXED PURE WHITE WITH HI-DEF CYAN AND WORKED THEM INTO THE SKIN WITH AN ILLAMASQUA BLUSHER BRUSH (WHICH I THINK IS THE PERFECT BRUSH FOR MAC PRO PAINT STICKS). I USED THE SAME LIGHT BLUE MIX TO SHADE THE CHIN AND JAWLINE. NORMALLY I WOULD USE A DARKER SHADING COLOR HERE, BUT BREAKING THE RULES IS KEY IN THIS LOOK; IT'S THE FREEDOM YOU GET WHEN YOU WORK AS AN ARTIST.

I APPLIED A WASH OF CHARTREUSE OVER THE ENTIRE EYE AREA ALL THE WAY UP TO THE BROWS USING A MAC 217 BLENDING BRUSH. I THEN FINISHED THE EYES WITH BLACK EYELINER USING MY FAVORITE THE FELINE FLICK IN PANTHER BY CHARLOTTE TILBURY. I ADDED TWO DOTS AT EACH END TO GIVE THE LINER UNIQUENESS AND PULLED THE LINE A THIRD OF THE WAY UNDERNEATH THE LOWER LASHES TO MAKE SOPHIA LOOK STERNER.

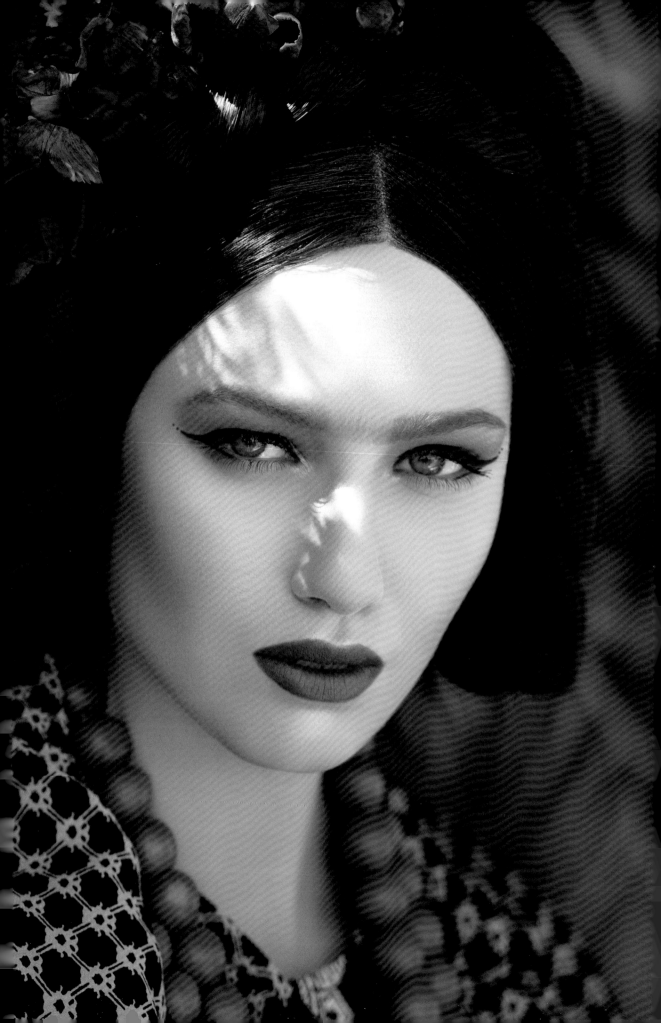

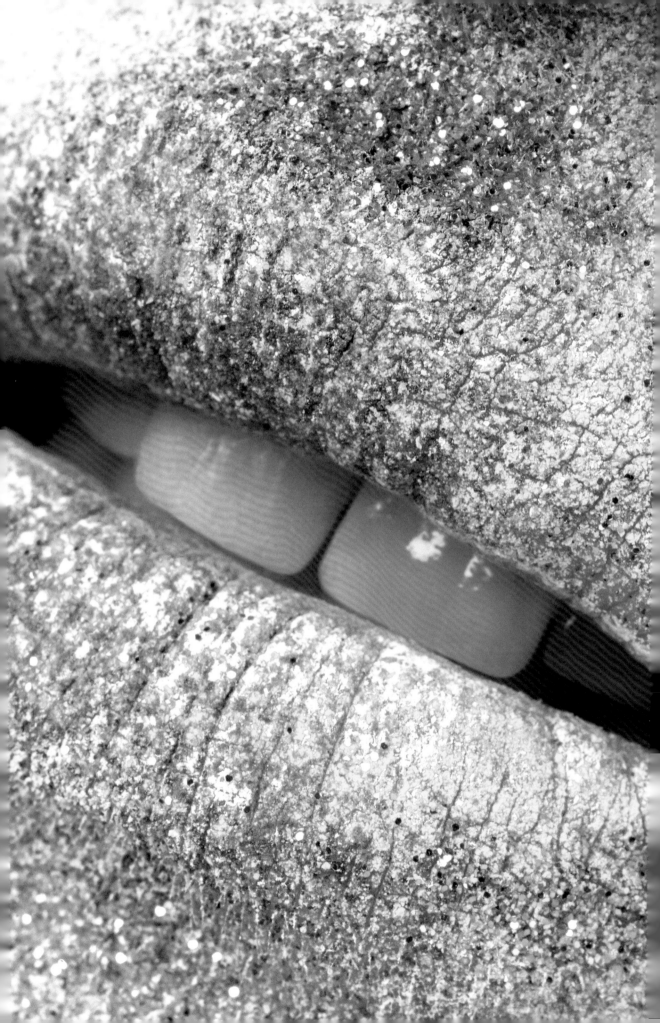

Fairy Dust

Children's chalk dusted onto the face creates a magical creature that seems to have come directly from the pages of a book of fairy tales.

PRIMER
Illamasqua Satin Primer applied in two layers.

SKIN
Crayola Drawing Chalk for +3 years (not sidewalk chalk) ground through a small kitchen sieve.

I first saw this technique, which involves dusting chalk through a fine sieve onto the face, at Loni Baur's amazing Color + Creme Academy in Germany, where she teaches the most incredible master classes to working makeup artists.

I started by priming the skin with <u>two layers</u> of <u>Illamasqua Satin Primer</u> to protect against staining. Then, to create the chalk hue, I first ground white chalk—my base color—through the sieve to cover most of the face. Next, I ground blue chalk to contour the hollow of the cheeks, above the temples, in the creases of the eyes, on the top of the forehead, and below the chin onto the jawline. I then used yellow chalk to set highlights on the eyelids, lips, and tops of the cheekbones. To finish, I added hints of purple and orange wherever I felt it needed more interest or depth.

While we were shooting, I kept adding bits of color ground through the sieve here and there—especially for the macro crops, which I tend to think need more rather than less detail.

Beware that if it is too warm in the room, the chalk melts into the skin and the texture is lost. It's for this reason that I probably prefer doing the same technique using loose pigment instead of chalk. If you do use chalk and feel the color fading into the skin, just reapply on top to freshen up the look.

Dark Romance

Darkly alluring, the goth girl has serious pulling power. With this look's plum-stained eyelids and a dark, pointed pout, only those with attitude need apply.

BASE
MAC Pro Full Coverage Foundations in NC15 and NC20 (mixed). Make Up For Ever HD Powder dusted across the T-zone.

CONTOUR
Illamasqua Powder Blusher in Disobey.

HIGHLIGHT
Laura Mercier Loose Setting Powder in Star Dust.

EYES
YSL Rouge Volupté Perle Lipstick in 112 Spellbinding Violet. MAC 217 Blending Brush. MAC 3 Lash single lashes in Medium and Long. Black mascara.

EYEBROWS
Inglot Brow Powders in 569 and 560.

LIPS
MAC Lip Pencil in Plum. Obsessive Compulsive Cosmetics Lip Tar in Metallic in Black Metal Dahlia as a base. YSL Rouge Volupté Perle in 112 Spellbinding Violet over the top.

What I love about goth culture is that both women and men express their personality and true nature through makeup. The uniquely romantic goth girl is a recurring theme for makeup artists, and I think it's because the essence of goth culture holds true for us as well. Makeup artists use makeup to tell the editorial story—we transform the model into a character and give her a totally new personality to run with.

My vampish interpretation here features two key elements: a pointy sultry lip and mystical, glossy eyes. I used MAC Lip Pencil in Plum to overdraw the lip into an exaggerated, pointy Cupid's bow. I then applied one coat of my favorite OCC Lip Tar: Metallic in Black Metal Dahlia. Once applied, however, I felt it looked too red, so I added a coat of the beautiful YSL Rouge Volupté Perle in 112 Spellbinding Violet over the top to darken.

Because I love making my products multitask, I used the same YSL lipstick to spread a thin coat of color over the eyelids using a MAC 217 Blending Brush. I then added lots of MAC 3 Lash single lashes in Medium and Long and finished with a coat of black mascara on the top and bottom lashes. Not every look needs eye shadow; sometimes the best results happen when you have fun experimenting with textures and using the products already in your kit to multitask.

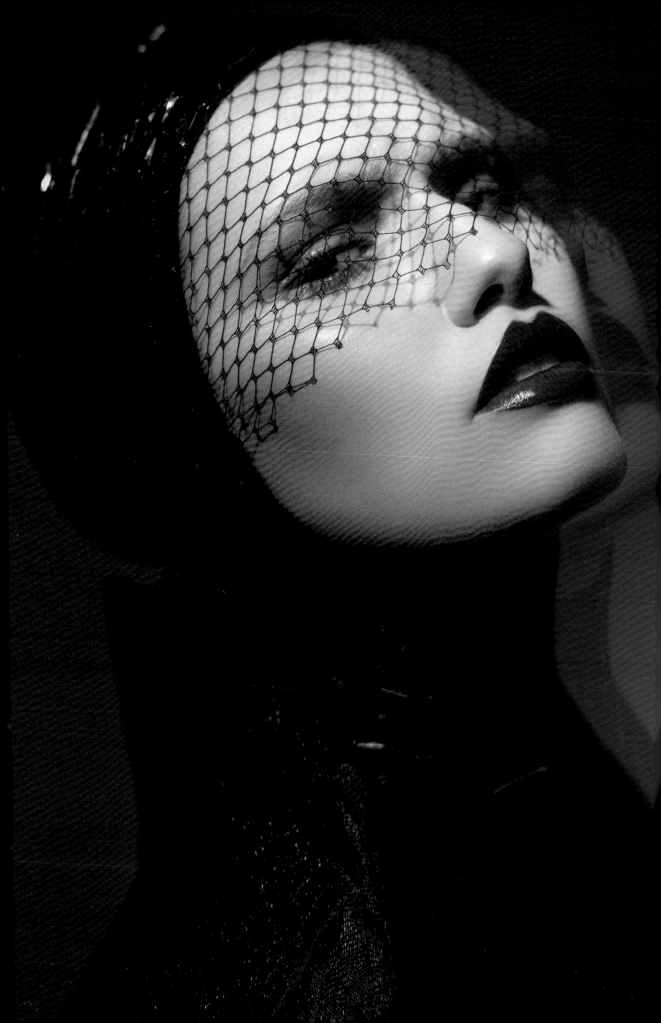

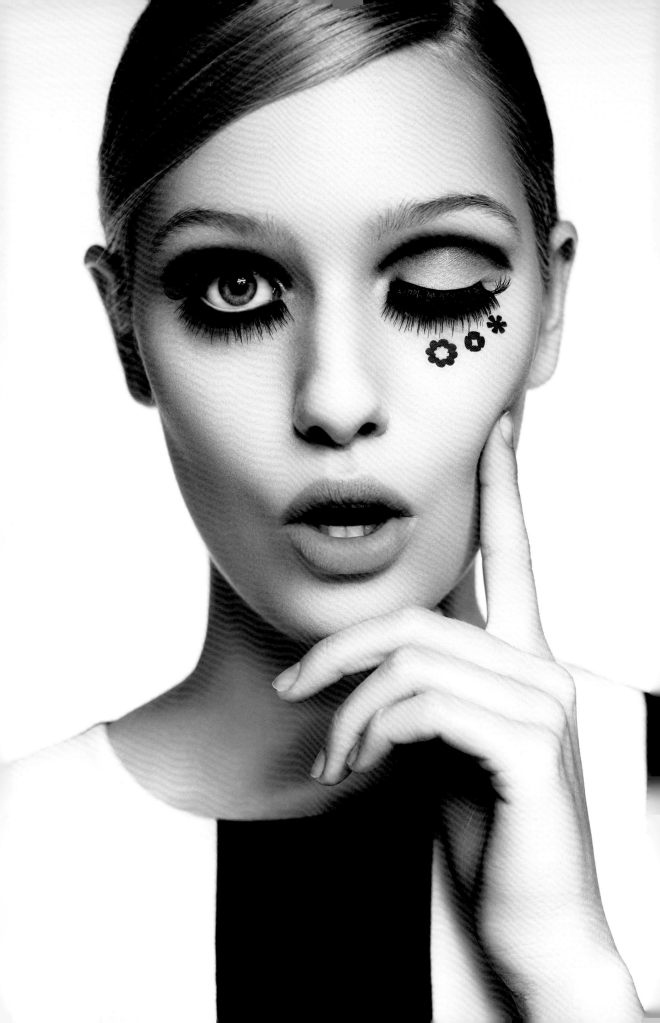

Blink!

TWIGGY'S BIG BABY-DOLL EYES STILL GET ALL THE ATTENTION. KEEP IT SLEEKLY MONOCHROMATIC AND PILE ON THE LASHES—ONE SET WILL NEVER BE ENOUGH.

BASE
MAC Pro Full Coverage Foundations in NC15 and NC20 (mixed). Make Up For Ever HD Powder to set.

CONTOUR
Illamasqua Powder Blusher in Disobey.

LIPS
MAC Lip Erase in Dim.

EYES
Illamasqua Pure Pigment in Breathe all over the eyelids. Kevyn Aucoin The Essential Eye Shadow in N° 110 Blackest Black to enhance the creases. MAC Fluidline in Blacktrack as eyeliner on the top lashes. MAC Eye Kohl in Fascinating on the waterlines. MAC 40 Lash and MAC 3 Lash on the top lashes. MAC 30 Lash single lashes in Medium and Short. Demi Wispy Lashes by Ardell.

FACE STICKERS
Face Lace by Phyllis Cohen in Floridots.

THE 1960s WERE SUCH A BEAUTIFUL ERA OF EXAGGERATED HAIR AND MAKEUP. IT WAS ALL ABOUT ENHANCING YOUR FAVORITE FEATURES AND MAKING A BOLD STATEMENT. THIS LOOK IS ALL ABOUT THE EYES. I USED ILLAMASQUA PURE PIGMENT IN BREATHE TO WASH A HINT OF SILVERY WHITE OVER THE EYELIDS AND TO HIGHLIGHT THE INNER CORNERS OF THE EYES. THEN, I ASKED SOPHIA TO KEEP HER EYES OPEN WHILE I ENHANCED THE HALF-MOON SHAPES JUST ABOVE THE CREASES OF HER EYES USING KEVYN AUCOIN'S AMAZING MATTE EYE SHADOW IN N° 110 BLACKEST BLACK. I THEN CREATED A BASE FOR THE FALSE EYELASHES BY DRAWING A SIMPLE BLACK EYELINER AT THE TOP LASH LINES USING MAC FLUIDLINE IN BLACKTRACK.

NEXT, I GLUED THE MAC 40 LASH TO THE TOP LASHES AND MAC 30 LASH SINGLE LASHES IN MEDIUM AND SHORT TO THE BOTTOM LASHES. I THOUGHT THIS WOULD BE PLENTY—BUT WHEN WE STARTED SHOOTING, ALTHOUGH IT LOOKED BEAUTIFUL, I FELT IT LACKED THE GUTSINESS SO TYPICAL OF '60s MAKEUP. TO RAMP THINGS UP SOME MORE, I APPLIED A SET OF MAC 3 LASH ON TOP OF THE OTHER SET OF LASHES AND A FULL SET OF DEMI WISPY LASHES BY ARDELL ON THE BOTTOM LASHES OVER THE ALREADY-GLUED SINGLE LASHES. THEN, TO ADD AN ELEMENT OF FUN, I STUCK THREE FACE LACE STICKERS FROM PHYLLIS COHEN'S BEAUTIFUL FLORIDOTS SET UNDER ONE OF THE EYES. MORE IS MORE IS MORE WHEN DOING '60s-INSPIRED MAKEUP—HOW COULD I FORGET?

THIS LOOK REMINDED ME THAT IT'S IMPORTANT TO ALWAYS BE BRAVE WHEN DOING MAKEUP AND TO COMMIT ONE HUNDRED PERCENT TO YOUR LOOK. DON'T HAVE YOUR EGO STOP YOU FROM ADMITTING A MISTAKE, AND NEVER BE SHY OF CHANGING THINGS IF YOU FEEL IT'S NOT LOOKING AMAZING ON CAMERA. THE FINAL IMAGE IS THE GOAL, SO ALWAYS DO WHATEVER YOU NEED TO DO TO MAKE YOUR PART PERFECT. THIS IMAGE IS SO STRIKING—I LOVE IT. BUT TO GET IT, WE NEEDED A LITTLE HELP IN POSTPRODUCTION—SOPHIA IS AN AMAZING MODEL, BUT EVEN SHE HAS HER FACIAL LIMITS! WE SHOT EACH OF SOPHIA'S POSES TWICE—ONE WITH HER EYES OPEN, THE OTHER WITH HER EYES CLOSED. WHAT YOU SEE HERE IS THE IMAGE WITH HER EYES OPEN, BUT WITH ONE OF HER CLOSED EYES INSERTED INTO THE IMAGE IN POSTPRODUCTION.

Black Magic

NOTHING IS MORE TRANSFORMATIVE OR EXCITING THAN
ALLOVER BODY PAINT. HERE, LILY WHITE IS TURNED BEAUTIFUL EBONY.
LIKE ANY GOOD MAGIC, IT'S ALL IN THE PREPARATION.

SKIN
Illamasqua Satin Matte Primer. MAC Pro Chromacake in Black Black applied with a MAC 187 Duo Fiber Brush and MAC 188 Small Duo Fiber Brush.

LIPS
Kryolan Clear Glitter Gel using an Illamasqua Lip Brush. Make Up For Ever Large Size Glitter in Black pressed onto the lips with a MAC 228 Mini Shader Brush.

CLEANSER
Johnson & Johnson Baby Soap.

I LOVE PAINTING MODELS BLACK—IT CHANGES EVERYTHING! THE FIRST TIME I DID THIS WAS FOR A "FASHION WARRIOR" EDITORIAL FOR *NOI.SE* MAGAZINE. THE MODEL WAS FROM UGANDA, AND ALL THE CLOTHES WERE BY ONE OF MY FAVORITE DESIGNERS AND GOOD FRIENDS, MICHAEL CINCO. MICHAEL ALSO DESIGNED THE DRESS SOPHIA WEARS HERE. UNLIKE MY GORGEOUS UGANDAN MODEL, SOPHIA HAS VERY LIGHT SKIN, SO I WAS EXTREMELY NERVOUS ABOUT PAINTING HER BLACK. TO PROTECT SOPHIA'S SKIN, I CAREFULLY APPLIED FOUR COATS OF ILLAMASQUA SATIN MATTE PRIMER (ON DARKER SKIN, I WOULD DO ONE OR TWO COATS) WHEREVER THE PAINT WAS GOING TO TOUCH HER SKIN. I REALLY TOOK MY TIME AND APPLIED PRIMER TO SOPHIA'S LIPS, FINGERS, AND NOSTRILS. I ALSO PRIMED MY OWN HANDS!

I USED MAC CHROMACAKE IN BLACK BLACK BECAUSE IT GIVES A MATTE FINISH AND PROVIDED A BEAUTIFUL CONTRAST TO MICHAEL CINCO'S BEAUTIFUL EMBELLISHED DRESS AND THE SHINY HAIR. TO ACTIVATE THE CHROMACAKE, I DIPPED THE TIP OF MY BRUSH IN WATER AND SWIRLED IT INTO THE CAKE. YOU NEED ONLY THE SMALLEST BIT OF WATER; TOO MUCH WILL CAUSE UNEVEN AND VISIBLE BRUSHSTROKES. IF THIS HAPPENS, DRY YOUR BRUSH OFF AND START AGAIN; YOU'LL SOON GET THE FEEL FOR THE AMOUNT OF WATER TO USE. I APPLIED THE BLACK PAINT TO SOPHIA'S LIMBS IN LONG, SWEEPING STROKES AND IN LITTLE SWIRLS ON HER FINGERS AND HANDS TO ENSURE PAINT WENT INTO ALL THE LITTLE LINES. I APPLIED TWO OR THREE COATS TO CREATE AN EVEN COVERAGE. TO FINISH, I CLEANED SOPHIA'S NAILS USING A WET WIPE WRAPPED AROUND A COTTON SWAB AND WAITED AT LEAST TWENTY MINUTES BEFORE TAKING ANY PROTECTIVE CLOTHING OFF.

CREATING CONTRAST IS IMPORTANT IN MAKEUP, SO I ADDED A SHINY GLITTER LIP. I FIRST APPLIED A THIN LAYER OF CLEAR KRYOLAN GLITTER GEL WITH AN ILLAMASQUA LIP BRUSH, THEN CAREFULLY PRESSED BLACK MAKE UP FOR EVER LARGE SIZE GLITTER INTO THE GEL WITH A MAC 228 BRUSH. A GREAT TIP FOR THIS TECHNIQUE IS TO AVOID PRESSING THE SAME AREA TWICE, WHICH WILL MATTIFY THE GLITTER. YOU'LL ALSO BE HAPPY TO KNOW THAT ALL THE PAINT WAS REMOVED FROM SOPHIA'S SKIN, USING JOHNSON & JOHNSON BABY SOAP, WITHOUT ANY STAINING. THE ILLAMASQUA PRIMER WORKED ITS MAGIC!

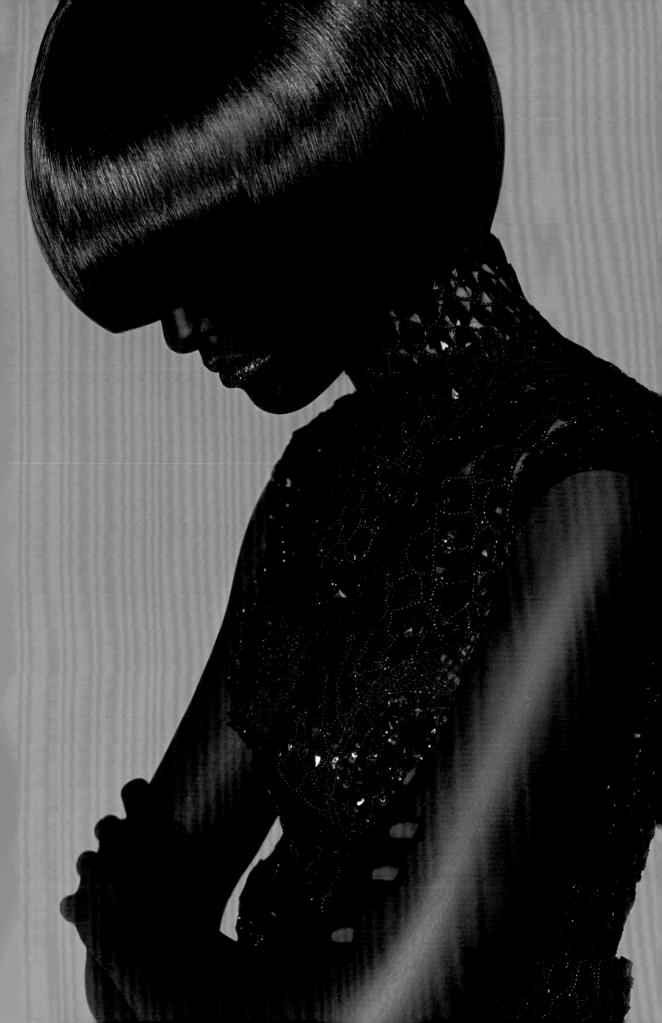

"Make your makeup more believable and organic by applying the highlight on the inner corners of the eyes and the Cupid's bow in an ever-so-slightly asymmetrical fashion."

Toni Malt

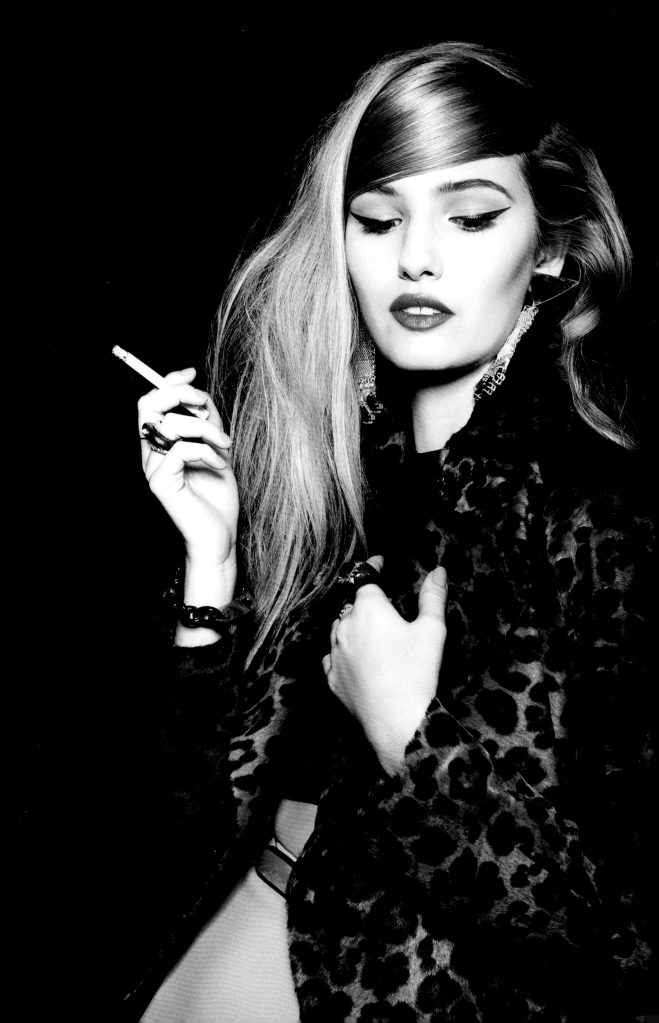

With the Band

A CLASSIC 1960S ROCK 'N' ROLL VIBE GETS A MODERN TWIST WITH A COLOR SHOT TO THE EYES, LIPS, AND NAILS. THIS IS A GIRL WHO KNOWS HOW TO ROCK IT.

BASE
Charlotte Tilbury Light Wonder Foundation in 2 Fair.
Charlotte Tilbury Airbrush Flawless Finish in 1 Fair to set.

CONTOUR
Illamasqua Powder Blusher in Disobey.

EYES
MAC Eye Shadow in Brun to contour the creases and below the lower lashes.
Illamasqua Pure Pigment in Breathe to highlight the inner corners.
Make Up For Ever Aqua Liner in 8 Iridescent Electric Purple to draw a slightly exaggerated eyeliner on the top lashes.
Illamasqua Sealing Gel mixed with Yaby Eye Shadow in pp064 Violet Crystal (from the Yaby World of Pearl Paint palette) to enhance the line.

EYEBROWS
MAC Eye Brows pencils in Lingering and Stud to enhance and strengthen the brows.
Inglot Brow Powders in 569 and 560 to finish.

LIPS
Lime Crime Lipstick in Beautiful Rocket.
MAC Matte mattifying cream over the top.

IT'S ALWAYS GOOD TO REASSESS YOUR COLOR CHOICE. ONCE I HAVE ROUGHLY WORKED OUT A LOOK FOR AN EDITORIAL, I LIKE TO ASK MYSELF, "COULD I MAKE MY LOOK STRONGER IF I USED A DIFFERENT COLOR?" "COULD I BE BRAVER?" "AM I REALLY COMMITTING TO THE LOOK, OR AM I PLAYING IT SAFE?"

HERE, SOPHIA AND I SHOT FOR ROLLING STONE MAGAZINE, AND THE FASHION EDITOR WAS LOOKING FOR A MODERN ROCK 'N' ROLL, 1960S LOOK. WHEN YOU THINK OF THE '60S, YOU IMMEDIATELY THINK OF BLACK EYELINER AND NUDE LIPS, SO TO MAKE THE LOOK A BIT MORE AMERICAN ROCK 'N' ROLL, I OPTED FOR A PURPLE EYELINER, ORANGE LIPS, AND PINK FINGERNAILS. I WANTED TO LET MY COLOR CHOICES REFLECT THAT THIS GIRL HAS GUTS AND IS A REAL ROLLING STONE KINDA GIRL.

SWAPPING BLACK EYELINER FOR A COLORED LINER (EVEN IF IT'S NOT A DRASTIC CHANGE—A DARK BLUE OR DARK PURPLE PERHAPS) WILL HAVE A BIG IMPACT ON YOUR LOOK. THERE ARE SO MANY EYELINERS AVAILABLE IN SUCH WONDERFUL COLORS TO TRY, BUT MY FAVORITES ARE DEFINITELY MAKE UP FOR EVER AQUA LINER, MAC SUPERSLICK LIQUID EYE LINER, AND MAC LIQUIDLAST LINER. AND A FANTASTIC WHITE EYELINER IS ILLAMASQUA PRECISION INK IN SCRIBE.

FOR THIS LOOK, I STARTED BY LINING THE EYES WITH MAKE UP FOR EVER AQUA LINER IN 8 IRIDESCENT ELECTRIC PURPLE. ONCE I'D APPLIED IT, HOWEVER, I FELT IT WAS TOO DARK, SO I LIGHTENED IT BY ADDING A MIX OF ILLAMASQUA SEALING GEL AND YABY EYE SHADOW IN PP064 VIOLET CRYSTAL ON TOP.

Precious Gems

Lips get sparklingly beautiful with super-dense turquoise glitter. The trick to capturing a great image is to keep the lips rounded and pile on the sparkles.

BASE
MAC Pro Full Coverage Foundation in NC15. Make Up For Ever HD Powder to set.

LIPS
MAC Chromagraphic Pencil in Hi-Def Cyan. Usha's Beauty Book 1. Sponge applicator.

Glitter lips are tricky and hard to get right for photography. Depending on the product you have used and on the photographer's lighting setup, it is sometimes impossible to get glitter lips to look great. I have done so many, and so many have looked strange! But I am so happy to have finally found a glitter product that looks amazing. It's Usha's Beauty Book 1, a palette of twenty-four highly dense glitter gel colors.

To create the lips, I used MAC Chromagraphic Pencil in Hi-Def Cyan to create a base over the entire lip. This was in case the gel let any lip color shine through. I then used a sponge applicator to carefully dab the glitter gel onto the lips. When you are finished, add the same amount again. The photographer's light seems to eat up glitter, leaving only half of the product visible in the image, so more is more! With so much product on, do remind your model not to smudge her lips during the shoot, and bring a straw for her to drink with.

This image is actually a happy accident. As you can see from the product list, no other makeup was used on the face—no eye makeup, no shading, no highlighting, nothing. I didn't even brush the eyebrows! We had originally intended to zoom in tightly on the lips, so I'd left the rest of Sophia's face bare. This shoot goes to show that you can never trust the photographer when he says he will crop in tight! Sylvio had temporarily zoomed out, and this is the result—just beautiful.

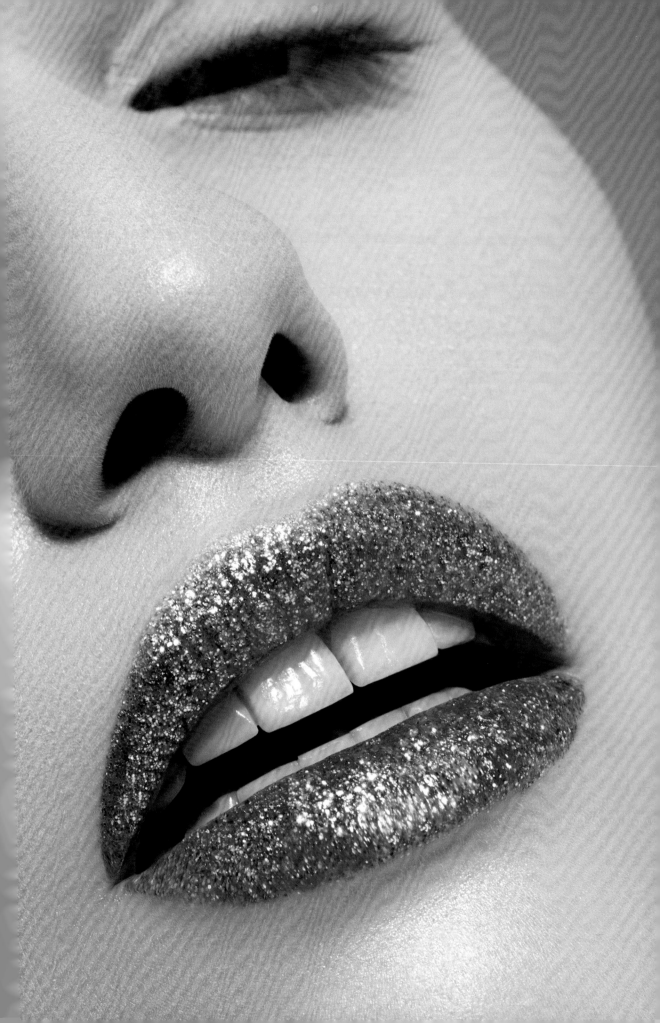

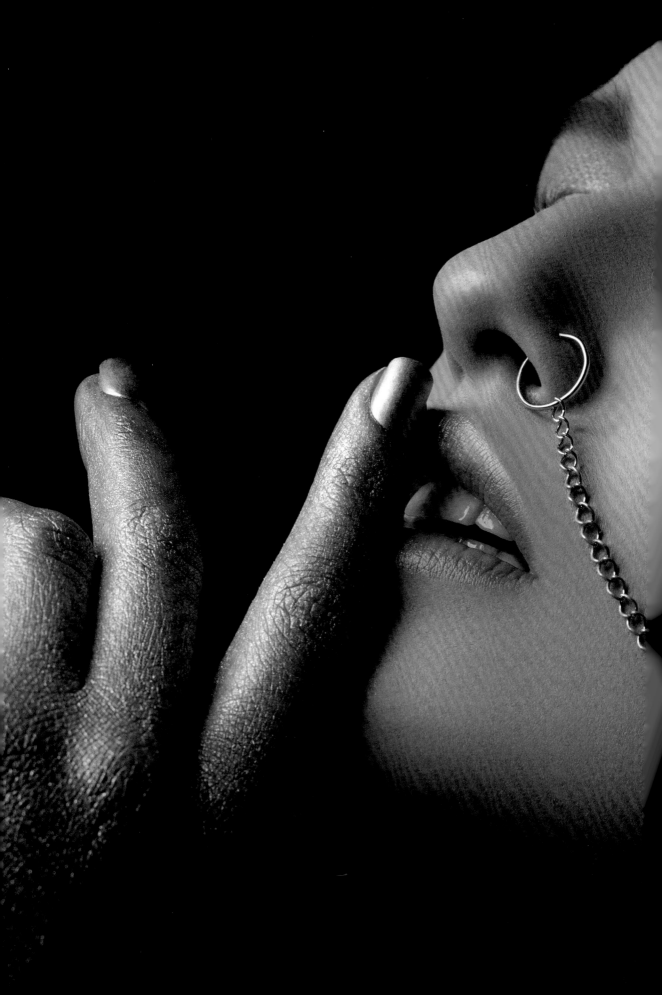

Heavy Metal

The best way to make an impact is to add the unexpected. Lids and hands get plated in silver, while a nose piercing adds toughness that's both luxe and undeniably hardcore.

BASE
Charlotte Tilbury Light Wonder Foundation in 4 Fair. Make Up For Ever HD Powder to set.

CONTOUR
MAC Powder Blusher in Taupe.

HIGHLIGHT
Skin N Nature Cookie Marble Blusher in 01 Rose.

EYES
MAC Eye Kohl in Smolder to tightline the eyes (or fill in between the lashes).
Kevyn Aucoin The Essential Eye Shadow in N° 110 Blackest Black to rim the outside of the eyes.
Make Up For Ever Wet Makeup in ARG Silver activated with a slightly wet MAC 217 Blending Brush.
Blend the edges quickly with a dry MAC 217 Blending Brush before the Wet Makeup dries.
A thin layer of Illamasqua Pure Pigment in Breathe over the silver to add shine and dimension.
Eylure Girls Aloud Lashes in Nicola on the top lash lines.
A coat of black mascara on the top and bottom lashes.

LIPS
Dior Addict Lipstick in Sand 414.

Make Up For Ever Wet Makeup is a wonderful product that comes in an amazing array of colors. Here, I have used it to add intensity to the eye makeup and to paint Sophia's hand metallic silver.

To create the eyes, I applied one layer of the Wet Makeup to each entire lid and up to the brow bones. Once the silver was dry, I enhanced the color with Illamasqua Pure Pigment in Breathe.

For the hand, I needed around five layers to get even coverage. It probably took me about fifteen minutes. I used silver nail polish on the nails, as the Wet Makeup doesn't adhere to fingernails. Make Up For Ever Wet Makeup does dry completely on skin, but I found it started to flake after Sophia brushed her hand against the jacket during the shoot. Thankfully, this product is easily removed from clothes with a wet wipe—a plus during a fashion shoot!

I really love the subtlety of the Make Up For Ever Wet Makeup in silver. However, when I want a really bold statement of almost molten metal, I opt for Kryolan Liquid Body Make-Up. It comes in silver, copper, bronze, and gold and gives a really beautiful, strong effect—it's definitely another favorite product!

Into the Blue

BEJEWELED LASHES, CRYSTAL EMBELLISHMENT, AND A MAGICAL MARINE-BLUE COMPLEXION—THE EFFECT IS WATERY AND MYSTICAL. SHE'S A CREATURE FROM THE DEEP.

BASE
Illamasqua Matt Satin Primer.
MAC Pro Paint Sticks in
Pure White, Hi-Def Cyan,
Marine Ultra, and Black Black.
Apply using Illamasqua
Blusher Brushes.

EYES
MAC Fluidline in Blacktrack
for the eyeliner on the top
lashes as a base.
Illamasqua Limited Edition
Lashes in Decadence.
DUO eyelash adhesive.

CRYSTALS
Various sizes of silver and blue
flat-back Swarovski crystals.
DUO eyelash adhesive.

I'VE SAID IT BEFORE AND I'LL SAY IT AGAIN: I LOVE MAC PRO PAINT STICKS! THEY ARE SUCH A FANTASTIC PRODUCT TO HAVE IN YOUR KIT BECAUSE THEY BLEND SO BEAUTIFULLY.

I USE THEM IN MANY DIFFERENT WAYS—MOST OFTEN AS EYE SHADOWS AND BLUSHES—BUT FOR THIS LOOK I USED MARINE ULTRA, PURE WHITE, AND HI-DEF CYAN AS A FOUNDATION.

TO APPLY, I FIRST PRIMED THE SKIN WITH ILLAMASQUA MATT SATIN PRIMER. I THEN CONTOURED THE FACE WITH THE DARKER MARINE ULTRA BEFORE TAKING THE COLOR LIGHTER TOWARD THE CENTER OF THE FACE WITH A MIXTURE OF PURE WHITE AND HI-DEF CYAN. ONCE WE STARTED SHOOTING, I DECIDED TO TAKE THE CONTOUR EVEN DARKER BY MIXING IN SOME BLACK BLACK PAINT STICK WITH THE MARINE ULTRA. THE PHOTOGRAPHER'S LIGHTING WAS SO BEAUTIFUL, AND WE WANTED TO GIVE THE IMPRESSION THAT THIS LOVELY FACE WAS CREATED OUT OF THE DARKNESS.

IF YOU LOOK AT THE BEHIND-THE-SCENES IMAGES, YOU'LL SEE THAT I ONLY PAINTED SOPHIA'S FACE HALFWAY. I KNEW WE WERE GOING TO SHOOT THIS IMAGE AT A CROP, AND AS WE SHOT IT TOWARD THE END OF THIS BOOK'S TWENTY-DAY SHOOT, SOPHIA'S SKIN HAD BECOME SO SENSITIVE TO BRUSHSTROKES THAT I WAS TRYING TO KEEP THINGS TO A MINIMUM.

ONCE THE FOUNDATION WAS DONE, I GLUED VARIOUS SIZES OF SILVER AND BLUE FLAT-BACK SWAROVSKI CRYSTALS TO THE FACE USING DUO EYELASH ADHESIVE. THIS TOOK ME ABOUT FORTY-FIVE MINUTES AS I NEEDED TO LET THE GLUE SET.

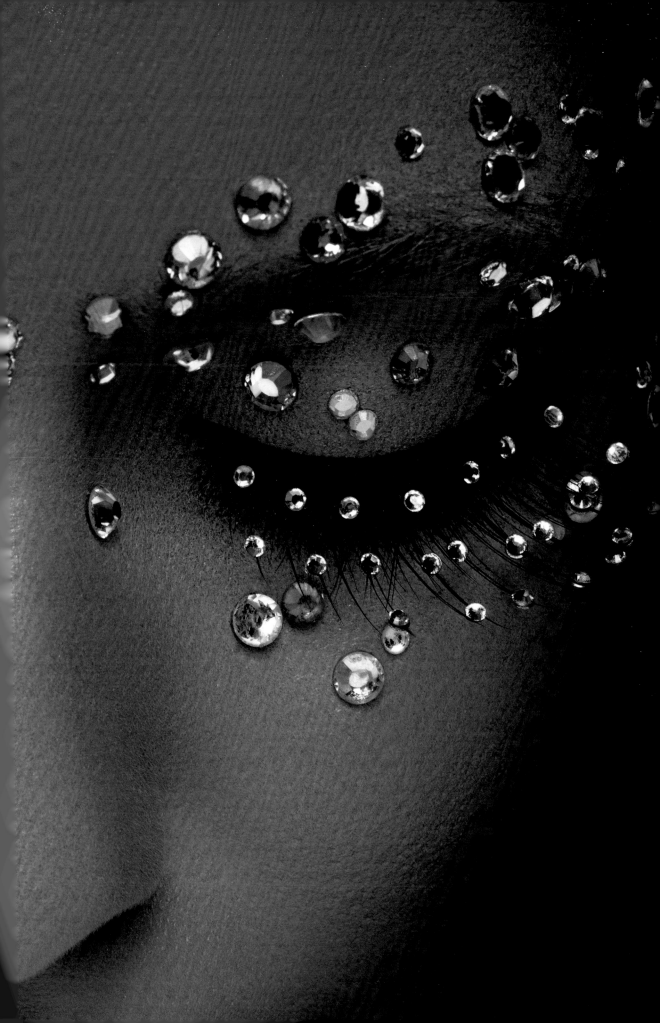

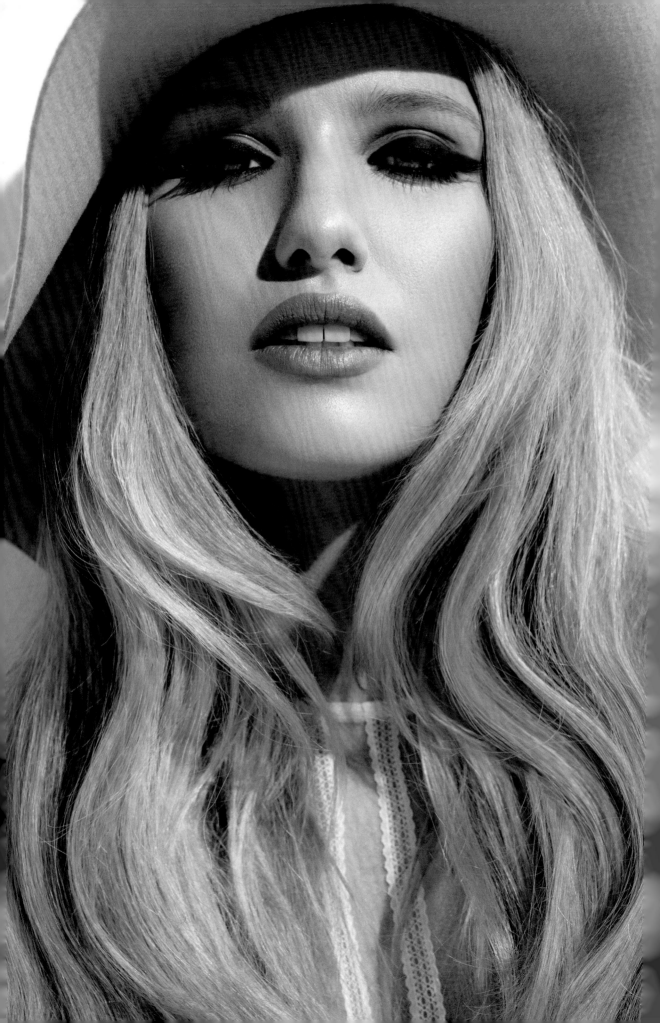

Belle du Jour

Brigitte Bardot's iconic style is still very much a part of today's lexicon. Thickly winged eyes, rounded lips, and hair for days: This is a beauty that will never go out of style.

FOUNDATION
MAC Pro Full Coverage Foundation in NC20.
Make Up For Ever HD Powder to set.

HIGHLIGHT
Skin N Nature Cookie Marble Blusher in 01 Rose.

CONTOUR
MAC Mineralize Skinfinish Natural in Medium Dark and Medium Deep (mixed).

EYES
Charlotte Tilbury Rock 'n' Kohl Iconic Liquid Eye Pencil in Bedroom Black, Kevyn Aucoin The Essential Eye Shadow in N° 110 Blackest Black.
Chanel 14 Contour Shadow Brush.
MAC Mineralize Skinfinish Natural in Medium Deep in the creases.
Eylure Girls Aloud Lashes in Nicola.
Black mascara.

EYEBROWS
Brushed and kept natural.

LIPS
MAC Lip Pencil in Subculture.
Rimmel Lasting Finish Lipstick by Kate Moss in 25.

Brigitte Bardot's trademark smoky winged eye and disheveled hair are an enduring inspiration for fashion and beauty editorials across the globe—and as Sophia already looks like Brigitte Bardot without makeup, she is the perfect model to re-create this legend of the 1950s and '60s.

An important element of creating these eyes is tightlining. That means I added Charlotte Tilbury Rock 'n' Kohl Iconic Liquid Eye Pencil in Bedroom Black to the waterlines of the eyes as well as between the top and bottom lashes. This pencil is just incredible because it will not move once it's applied, and it's truly black—not grayish or bluish like so many other black pencils.

I used the same eye pencil to frame the eyes and create a slight winged effect straight out to the sides, rather than upward as in a flick. I then softened the shape by applying Kevyn Aucoin The Essential Eye Shadow in N° 110 Blackest Black over the pencil and blended the edges with a Chanel 14 Contour Shadow Brush. The shadow will get rid of any harsh lines and give the look that slightly messy style typical of Bardot. To emphasize the winged-eye effect, I glued a pair of Eylure Girls Aloud Lashes in Nicola on top, then added heaps of black mascara to both the top and bottom lashes.

I sculpted the face and the creases of the eyes using MAC Mineralize Skinfinish Natural in Medium Dark and Medium Deep and finished with Rimmel Lipstick by Kate Moss in 25. Bardot had these beautiful, very rounded lips, so I applied the lipstick in one big round sweep across the top lip, totally ignoring the Cupid's bow. Wow, we were so lucky that Sophia has a gap in her teeth—she looks almost identical to Brigitte Bardot with this makeup.

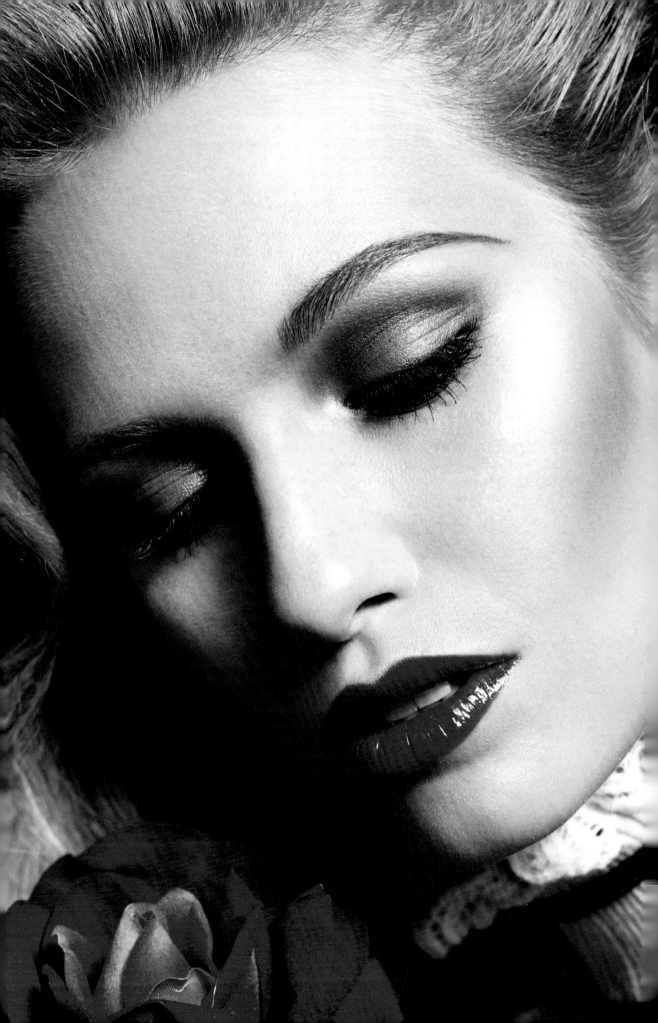

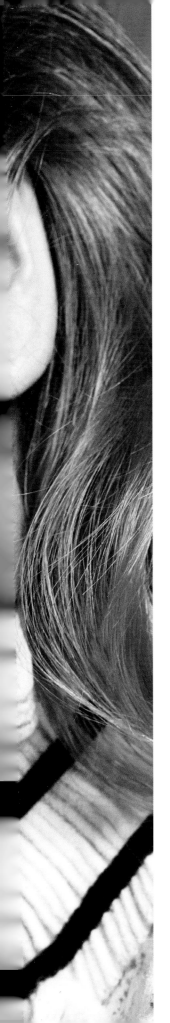

Into the Light

A CHANGE IN THE PHOTOGRAPHER'S LIGHTING CAN DRAMATICALLY ALTER THE FINAL IMAGE. HERE, THE MAKEUP LOOK TAKES ON TWO TOTALLY DIFFERENT MOODS.

All Chanel products are from the Chanel Méditerranée Summer 2015 Makeup Collection and Collection Plumes Précieuses de Chanel.

BASE
A very small amount of Chanel Vitalumière Aqua in 20 Beige applied with a Chanel Foundation Brush #6 and a Make Up For Ever Powder Brush in Medium 126.

CONTOUR
Chanel Lumière d'Été Illuminating Powder.

HIGHLIGHT
Chanel Limited Edition Camelia de Plumes Highlighting Powder.

EYES
Chanel Limited Edition Stylo Eyeshadow in 147 Caroube applied as a soft, smoky eye. Chanel Écriture de Chanel Eyeliner Pen in 10 Noir to intensify the upper lash lines. Chanel Stylo Yeux Waterproof Long-Lasting Eyeliner in 88 Noir Intense applied to the upper and lower waterlines. Chanel Illusion D'Ombre Long Wear Luminous Eyeshadow in 81 Fantasme applied in the inner corners to highlight. Chanel Le Volume de Chanel Waterproof Mascara in 10 Noir on the top and bottom lashes.

EYEBROWS
Le Sourcil de Chanel Perfect Brows.

LIPS
Chanel Rouge Coco Ultra Hydrating Lip Colour in 444 Gabrielle. Chanel Lèvres Scintillantes Glossimer lip gloss in 457 Allegria.

LIGHT IS EVERYTHING FOR A MAKEUP ARTIST, BOTH IN THE APPLICATION PROCESS AND IN TRANSLATING THE EDITORIAL STORY.

NATURAL SUNLIGHT IS THE BEST LIGHT TO APPLY MAKEUP, BUT RARELY AM I ABLE TO MAKE USE OF IT. CALL TIMES ARE OFTEN SO EARLY THAT THERE ISN'T A SINGLE RAY OF SUNLIGHT. I STRUGGLED WITH THIS FOR YEARS AND OFTEN HAD TO DO MAJOR LAST-MINUTE CORRECTIONS ON SET ONCE THE LIGHT TEST WAS DONE. BUT NO MORE! NOW I ARRIVE ON LOCATION EQUIPPED WITH MY OWN LIGHT SOURCES. I LOVE MY KEY LIGHT KIT BY TML. IT IS A DIMMABLE, DAYLIGHT-BALANCED LIGHT ON A TRIPOD THAT GIVES THE PERFECT LIGHT FOR MAKEUP APPLICATION AND HELPS KEEP ON-SET CORRECTIONS TO A MINIMUM. I ALSO CARRY A HEADLAMP FOR BACKSTAGE LINEUP TOUCH-UPS AND PUT A WHITE CAPE ON MY MODEL DURING APPLICATION TO REFLECT LIGHT BACK ONTO THE FACE.

IT IS IMPORTANT THAT A MAKEUP ARTIST UNDERSTAND THE BASICS OF LIGHTING AND HOW THIS AFFECTS MAKEUP; OFTEN I'LL NEED TO ADJUST MY MAKEUP TO FIT THE PHOTOGRAPHER'S LIGHTING MOOD. WHEN SHOOTING IN DAYLIGHT, I TEND TO USE MUCH LESS PRODUCT OVERALL AS NATURAL LIGHT

Into the Light

(continued)

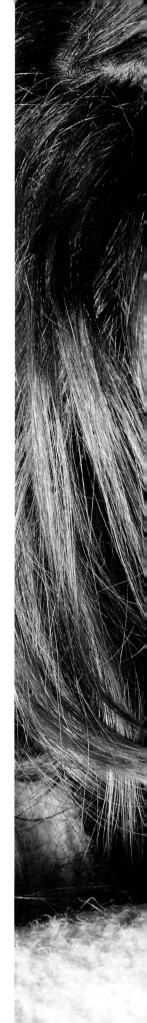

IS NOT VERY FORGIVING—YOU SEE EXACTLY WHAT'S THERE—AND MAKEUP SHOULD LOOK ORGANIC AND REAL. WHEN THE PHOTOGRAPHER SHOOTS WITH BIG HMI LIGHTS, I OFTEN FIND MYSELF OVEREMPHASIZING THE DEWINESS OF THE SKIN OR OVERDOING THE HIGHLIGHTS TO KEEP THE SKIN LOOKING ALIVE AND TO PREVENT IT FROM LOOKING MATTE. THEN THERE ARE TIMES WHEN THE PHOTOGRAPHER REALLY PUMPS UP THE POWER ON THE LIGHTS— NO MATTER WHAT IS USED AS A BASE, THE SKIN WILL OFTEN LOOK SWEATY UNDER SUCH BRIGHT LIGHT. FOR THESE SHOOTS I KEEP MY MAKE UP FOR EVER HD POWDER NEARBY TO CONTROL THE SHINE.

THE MAKEUP ARTIST'S APPLICATION DELIVERS THE PLOT OF A BEAUTY EDITORIAL STORY, BUT THE PHOTOGRAPHER'S LIGHT WILL ALWAYS DECIDE HOW THE STORY WILL BE TOLD. LOOK AT THESE TWO IMAGES OF SOPHIA. HER MAKEUP IS EXACTLY THE SAME IN EACH PHOTOGRAPH, BUT THEY APPEAR VASTLY DIFFERENT BECAUSE THE PHOTOGRAPHER HAS CHANGED THE LIGHTING SETUP (THE HAIR AND CLOTHES HAVE BEEN CHANGED TOO). NOTICE HOW DRAMATICALLY THE COLOR OF HER SKIN HAS CHANGED AND HOW DIFFERENT THE LIPSTICK COLOR APPEARS. BUT PERHAPS THE MOST IMPORTANT ELEMENT IS THE CHANGE IN MOOD: THE LOOK HAS GONE FROM SOMETHING SUBDUED AND STYLIZED TO A MORE MODERN, YOUNGER, FRESHER FEEL.

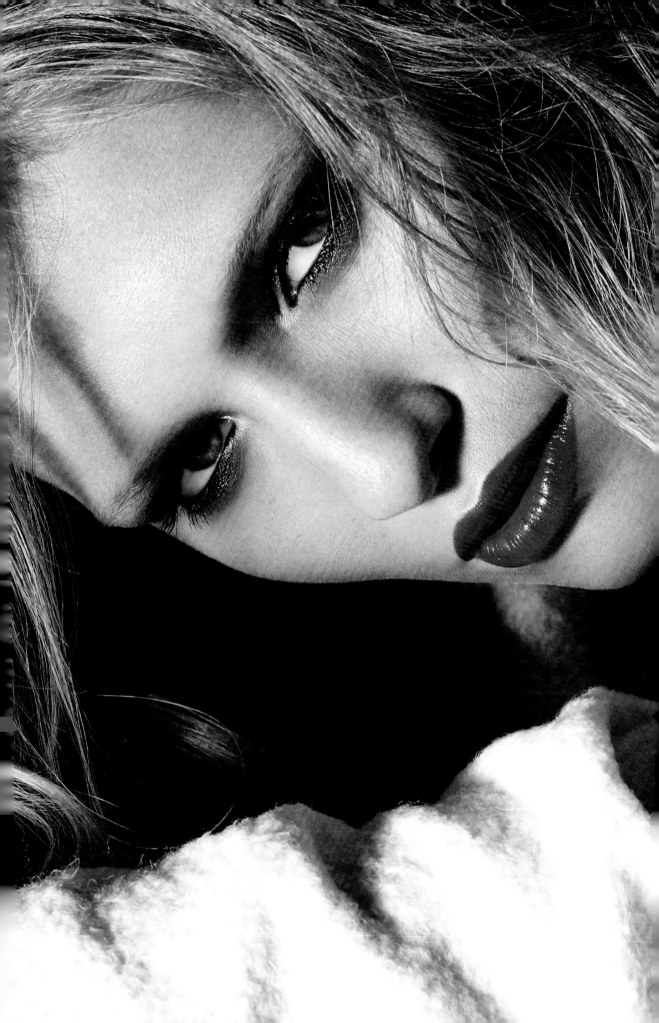

Ray of Light

Natural lighting and dramatic styling give this look its makeup cues. Pairing opposing shades on the color wheel creates balance, while careful blending gives plenty of romantic softness.

BASE
Charlotte Tilbury Light Wonder Foundation in 2 Fair.

CONTOUR
Charlotte Tilbury Filmstar Bronze & Glow enhanced with a touch of Illamasqua Bronzer in Writhe.

HIGHLIGHT
Laura Mercier Face Illuminator in Spellbound.

Color theory is such an exciting subject for makeup artists. Elegance, warmth, coldness, tranquility, vibrancy...it can all be created through color.

All makeup artists rely on the color wheel when using correctors. We all know that opposing colors cancel each other out—that orangey concealers cancel out bluish under-eye circles and green-pigmented concealers camouflage redness. But color theory can also be used in all facets of makeup color. When shooting beauty or fashion editorials, I apply the principles of color theory and consider how my work can add to the final images. I look at the set, the clothes, and the accessories. I check if any colored gels are being used over the lights or if any special treatments will be applied to the images in postproduction. This helps me understand how my makeup will be shot and what factors will influence it.

I like to think in terms of complementary and analogous (or adjacent) colors. Analogous colors (side-by-side colors) on the color wheel create a very Zen and harmonious feel. Imagine a model in a vibrant green suit against the dark blue backdrop of the New York streets with beautiful bronzed, nude makeup. Green—blue—yellow/orange; they're all right next to each other on the color wheel. Had the model worn a vibrant purple outfit, maybe

EYES

Tom Ford Eye Color Quad 02 Cognac Sable (the golden beige and light brown shades) to create a light, contoured wash of color over the lids and below the eyes.

Make Up For Ever Metal Powders in 1 Sunflower Gold and 3 Honey Gold softly blended together over the eyelids and underneath the eyes to achieve a golden orange.

Illamasqua Pure Pigment in Breathe and Charlotte Tilbury Bar of Gold blended and applied to the middle of the lids and at the inner corners of the eyes to highlight.

Chanel Écriture de Chanel Eyeliner Pen in 10 Noir to create a thin eyeliner at the base of the lashes.

One coat of black mascara on the top and bottom lashes.

EYEBROWS

Inglot Brow Powders in 569 and 560.

LIPS

Mix Vaseline with the same pigment used on the eyes to create a matching lipstick.

A STARK GLOSSY RED LIP WOULD HAVE BEEN SENSATIONAL. UNDERSTANDING THE COLOR WHEEL CAN BE A VERY POWERFUL TOOL. OF COURSE, DON'T FORGET THAT RULES CAN ALWAYS BE BROKEN!

WE SHOT THIS IMAGE USING ONLY THE DAYLIGHT THAT WAS AVAILABLE IN OUR BEAUTIFUL STUDIO. TO COMPLEMENT THE COOL BLUE-TINTED BACKGROUND, I BLENDED A LOT OF BRONZY COLORS OVER THE FOUNDATION TO GIVE SOPHIA'S ALABASTER SKIN WARMTH. STARTING WITH CHARLOTTE TILBURY FILMSTAR BRONZE & GLOW, I BOOSTED THE COLOR WITH ILLAMASQUA BRONZER IN WRITHE. I INTRODUCED A LOT OF ORANGEY-BROWN AND ORANGEY-GOLD COLORS TO THE EYES AND LIPS, MAKING SURE EVERYTHING WAS REALLY SOFT AND PERFECTLY BLENDED TO COMPLEMENT THE VERY PURE FEEL OF THE ORCHID HEADPIECE. YOU MIGHT BE THINKING THAT THE BACKGROUND ISN'T REALLY BLUE AND THE MAKEUP ISN'T REALLY ORANGE, BUT IT DOESN'T NEED TO BE. COLOR THEORY WORKS EVEN IN ABSTRACT FORM. THERE IS A BLUISH FEEL TO THE BACKGROUND AND AN ORANGEY FEEL TO THE MAKEUP.

THESE COMPLEMENTARY FEELINGS OF COLOR MAKE A VISUAL CONTRAST AND APPEAR STRONGER WHEN PLACED AGAINST EACH OTHER. THAT'S WHY THIS IMAGE WORKS.

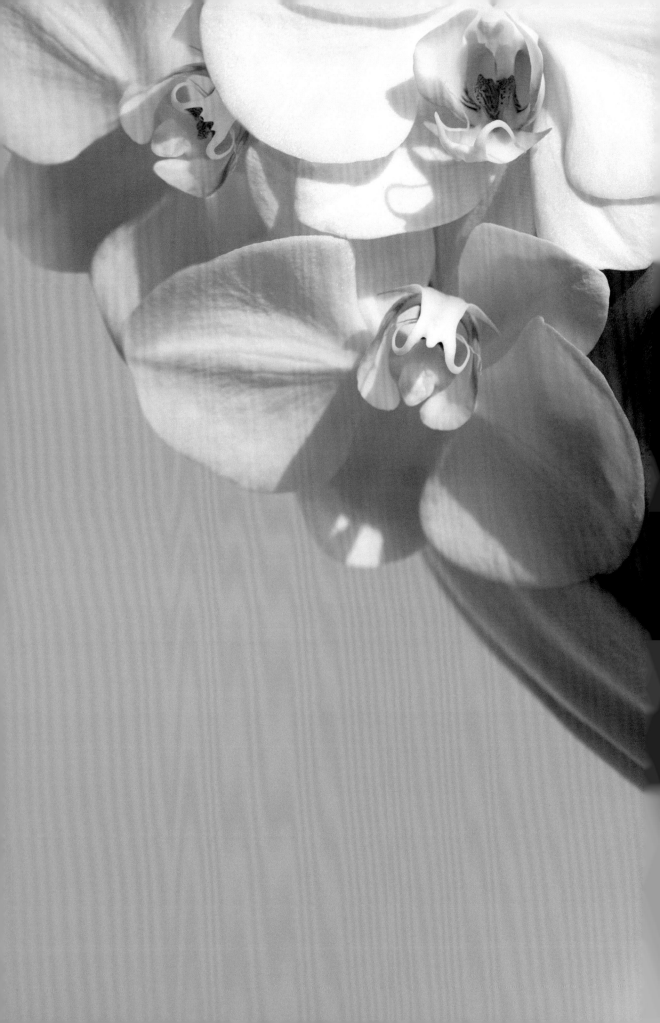

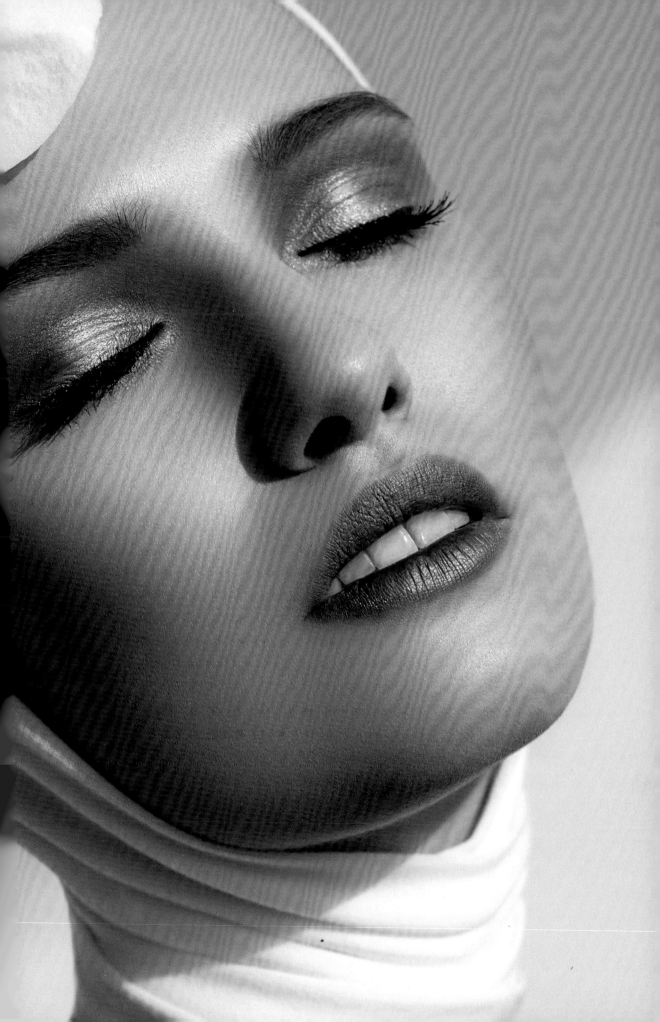

Body Beautiful

An athletic shoot requires an allover body glow—add water, and makeup needs to be water resistant, too. This glowing look is as resilient as it is fun.

BASE
MAC Pro Full Coverage Foundation in NW30.
Chanel Poudre Signée de Chanel Illuminating Powder to set.

CONTOUR
Illamasqua Powder Blusher in Disobey.

BLUSH
Scott Barnes Body Bling Shimmering Body Lotion in Platinum.

LIPS
Lime Crime Opaque Lipstick in D'Lilac mixed with a small amount of MAC Lipsticks in Violetta and Show Orchid to warm up the color.

EYES
Illamasqua Powder Blusher in Disobey to contour the creases.
Illamasqua Powder Blusher in Disobey under the lower lashes.
Illamasqua Pure Pigment in Breathe in the inner corners.
MAC Eye Kohl in Fascinating on the waterlines.
Black waterproof mascara on the top and bottom lashes.

SKIN
Scott Barnes Body Bling Shimmering Body Lotion in Platinum.

Oh, don't we all wish we had this beautiful California-girl tan all year long! I initially wanted to use Ben Nye's Bronzing Body Tint to achieve Sophia's beautiful allover body tan. This tint would have made Sophia's skin tone four to six shades darker with a single application. It's a great product if you want to achieve a realistic skin tone change. If you layer it, it's possible to achieve Kate Moss's famous Roberto Cavalli Eyewear campaign bronzed look, which was created by makeup artist Charlotte Tilbury and shot by famed photography duo Mert and Marcus.

The problem I faced for this shoot was that, to make the Ben Nye Bronzing Body Tint water resistant, I would need to use Ben Nye's Final Seal spray over the top, and this would have matted down the skin—the opposite of the golden glow I wanted to achieve. In the end, I used two layers of Scott Barnes Body Bling Shimmering Body Lotion in Platinum to create Sophia's beautiful bronzed look. I applied it to all exposed skin with my hands, taking my time and blending well. It took me about half an hour to tan the legs, stomach, back, arms, and décolletage. I also applied a little bit of the Body Bling on the eyes and cheeks to tie in all of Sophia's glowing skin with the makeup.

As a professional model, Sophia had never been this tanned in her life. Because we shoot winter editorials in the summer and summer editorials in the winter, Sophia follows her agency's advice and stays rather pale throughout the year. You can only imagine how happy she was running around the studio in her little sports outfit with this gorgeous tan. It's amazing how happy a tan can make someone.

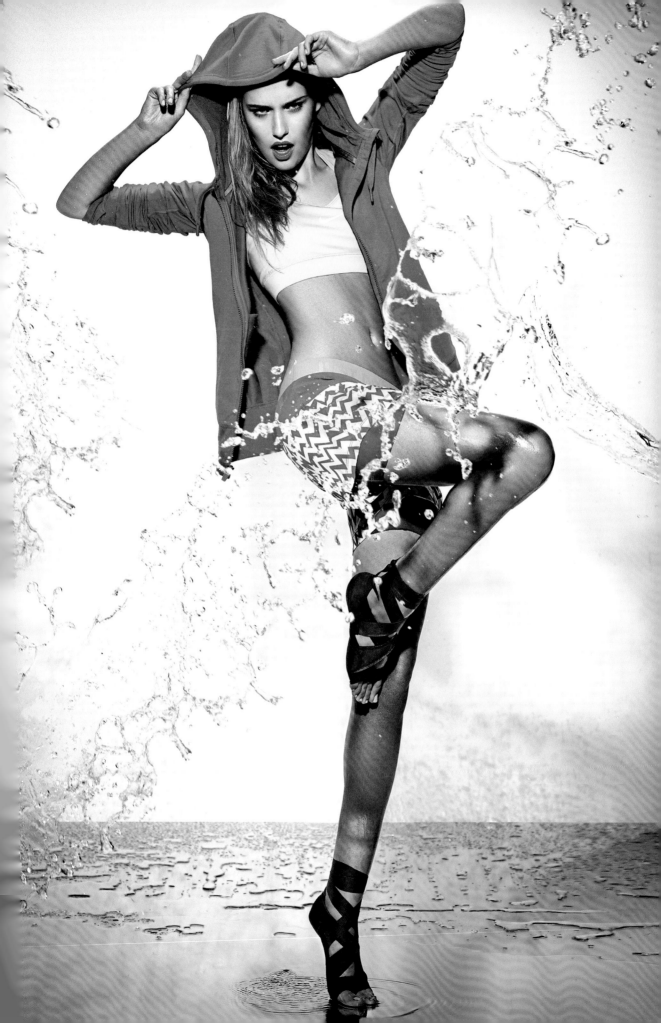

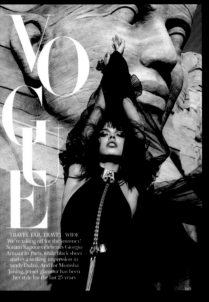
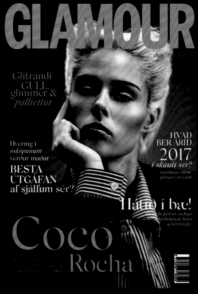
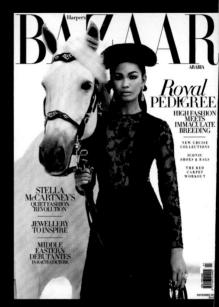
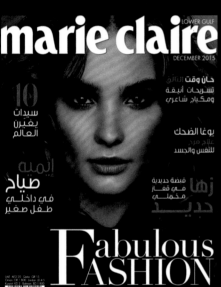
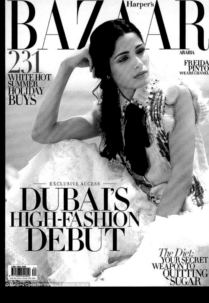
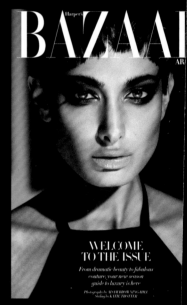
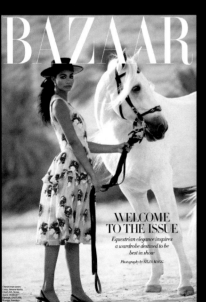
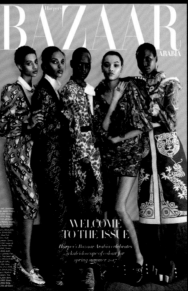
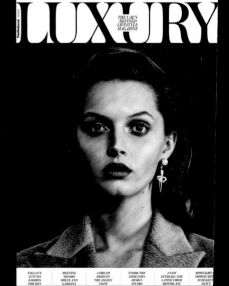

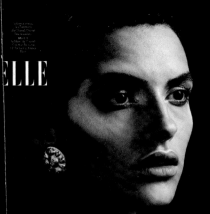

ELLE

fashion

On our agenda this February, smoking outfits that have never looked sexier, embroideries and dazzling dresses that seduce the modern-day princess, new accessories emerge from their lairs, and jewellery become talismans.

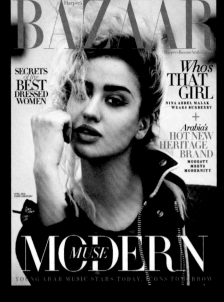

Harper's
BAZAAR

SECRETS of the BEST DRESSED WOMEN

Who's THAT GIRL
NINA ABDEL MALAK WEARS BURBERRY

+ *Arabia's* HOT NEW HERITAGE BRAND
MODESTY MEETS MODERNITY

MODERN *MUSE*

YOUNG ARAB MUSIC STARS TODAY, ICONS TOMORROW

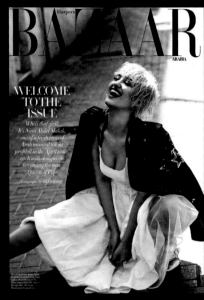

Harper's
BAZAAR
ARABIA

WELCOME TO THE ISSUE

Who's that girl? It's Nina Abdel Malak, one of a fresh crop of Arab musical talent profiled in the April issue, each with designs on becoming the new Queen of Pop

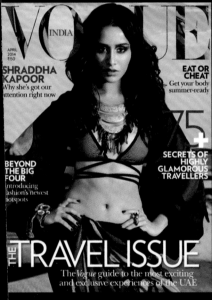

VOGUE
INDIA

APRIL 2014 ₹150

SHRADDHA KAPOOR
Why she's got our attention right now

EAT OR CHEAT
Get your body summer-ready

75+
SECRETS OF HIGHLY GLAMOROUS TRAVELLERS

BEYOND THE BIG FOUR
Introducing fashion's newest hotspots

THE TRAVEL ISSUE
The *Vogue* guide to the most exciting and exclusive experiences of the UAE

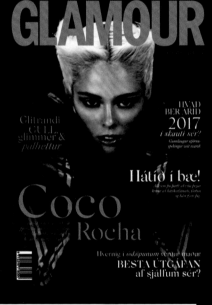

GLAMOUR

Glitrandi GULL glimmer & *pallettur*

HVAD BER ARID 2017
i skaut ser?
Gamlangar stjörnu spekingar vit varah

Hátió í bæ!

Coco Rocha

Hvernig i osköpunum verdur madur
BESTA ÚTGÁFAN
af sjálfum sér?

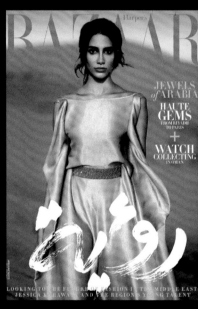

Harper's
BAZAAR

JEWELS of ARABIA
HAUTE GEMS FROM RIYADH TO PARIS

+ WATCH COLLECTING IN OMAN

رؤية

LOOKING TO THE FUTURE OF FASHION IN THE MIDDLE EAST
JESSICA K MAWAD AND THE REGION'S YOUNG TALENT

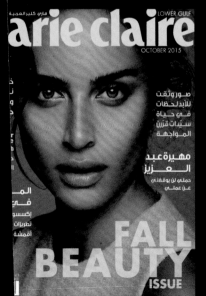

marie claire
LOWER GULF

OCTOBER 2015

صورتوقت للبدعلحظات في حياة سيدات قرن المواجهة

مهيرة عبد العزيز حملي لن يوقفني عن عملي

FALL BEAUTY
ISSUE

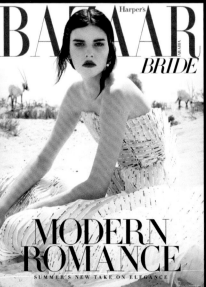

Harper's
BAZAAR
ARABIA
BRIDE

MODERN ROMANCE
SUMMER'S NEW TAKE ON ELEGANCE

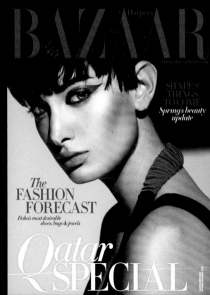

Harper's
BAZAAR

SHAPE of THINGS TO COME
Spring's beauty update

The FASHION FORECAST
Doha's most desirable shoes, bags & jewels

Qatar SPECIAL

Toni on the Making of *Transform*

WHERE DID THE CONCEPT OF ONE MODEL/SIXTY LOOKS COME FROM?
Rather than picking the "right" model for a particular look, this book demonstrates how any look can be achieved regardless of the face you're working on. All it takes is skill and knowledge. Hone your technique and you can do anything.

HAS LIVING AND WORKING IN DUBAI INFLUENCED THE BOOK?
Dubai is a developing fashion hub, so working there has had its challenges. When I started working ten years ago, the market mostly revolved around commercial campaigns, so there were very few agencies with editorial models. I found myself working with the same five editorial models again and again. I had no choice but to transform these few girls into whatever editorial creature I wanted them to be on that particular day. That is definitely where the inspiration for the book came from.

WHY SIXTY MAKEUP LOOKS?
Sixty looks was probably slightly overdoing it! But I wouldn't do less if I were to do it again. I felt I could only demonstrate the importance of skill and technique by showcasing how far makeup can be pushed. I wanted to overdo it to prove in how many exciting ways a makeup artist can add to a shoot.

WHERE DID YOU GET YOUR INSPIRATION?
I spent a lot of time with my fashion stylist developing each look. Sometimes the inspiration came from the clothes the designers supplied us; sometimes it came from current or recurring trends that we'd fallen in love with over the years. Other looks demonstrate learned-on-the-job skills that aren't taught in makeup school. And then there are the looks that are inspired purely by amazing product.

WHAT IS IT ABOUT YOUR MODEL SOPHIA THAT MADE HER PERFECT FOR TRANSFORM?
A beautiful face is important, but it's character that inspires me as a makeup artist. Sophia is undeniably beautiful, with her classic face structure, to-die-for cheekbones, cheeky gapped front teeth, full lips, and sky blue eyes. But what struck me about Sophia when I first met her was her boldness and magnetic charm. Our first shoot together involved my turning Sophia's skin alabaster white and changing her blonde hair burgundy red with

corkscrew curls (see the Fade to White look). After two hours, Sophia walked on set looking like a mythical creature. I was mesmerized by her beauty and ability to change into another character. I knew right then that she would be perfect.

How long did it take to create TRANSFORM?

I spent two years developing the book's content and direction. I was constantly writing down ideas, and I spent a lot of time researching and reading every bit of educational material I could get my hands on. I then spent another two weeks working out the shot list for the twenty-day shoot.

How did you choose your team?

Choosing my team members was probably the easiest part of creating this book. I have worked many times with each of them on fashion editorials, and I love their style and can-do attitude. I respect them all greatly; some of my happiest moments have been with this team in the studio creating this book.

Where was TRANSFORM created?

The whole book was created in and around Dubai. We set up camp in the gorgeous Hotcold Studio. With its beautiful natural daylight, the studio allowed us great flexibility with lighting and sets. Occasionally, we also shot in Dubai's old industrial district, which has some fantastic outdoor locations. We were in the studio day and night for twenty days, so it became like a second home.

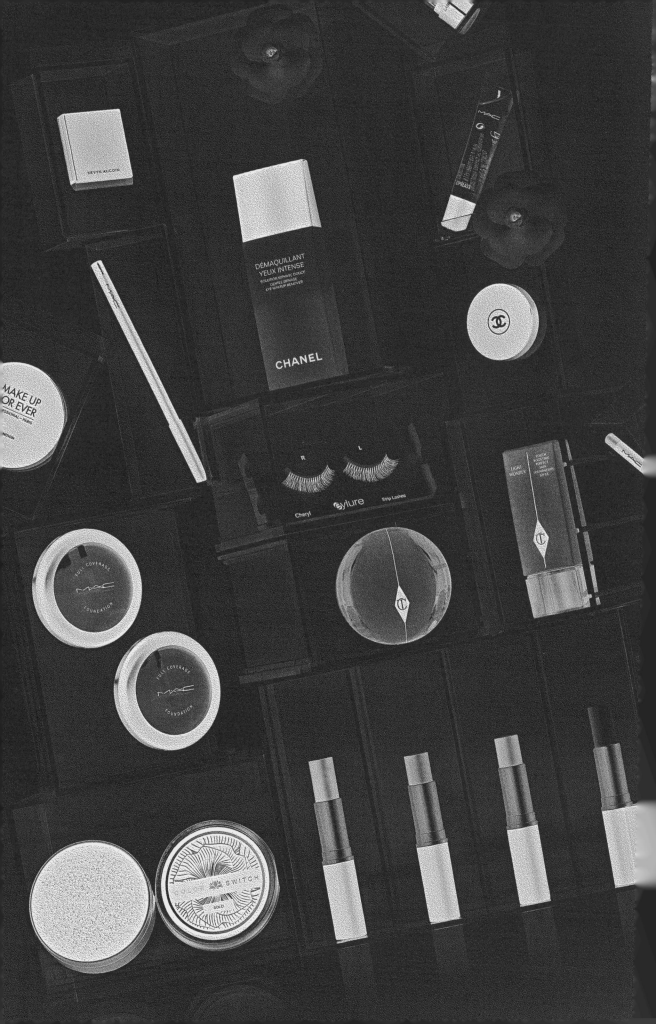

INSIDE TONI'S KIT

The Secrets of Toni's Makeup Kit

CHARLOTTE TILBURY CHARLOTTE'S MAGIC CREAM — This moisturizer by Charlotte Tilbury truly is magical. It preps the face beautifully and keeps skin hydrated throughout a long shoot day. It's so good that models often walk off a shoot with better-looking skin than when they first walked in that morning.

CHANEL DÉMAQUILLANT YEUX INTENSE EYE MAKEUP REMOVER — A beauty shoot can require up to seven partial or full makeup changes. This eye makeup remover by Chanel removes makeup quickly yet keeps skin nourished and prepped for the next makeup application. I prefer spending time applying makeup, not removing it.

CHARLOTTE TILBURY LIGHT WONDER FOUNDATION — My go-to foundation! Skin should still look like skin, and this lightweight next-generation foundation achieves the perfect coverage. It creates modern, luminous skin that stays hydrated even after a long day of shooting.

MAC PRO FULL COVERAGE FOUNDATION — I use this foundation for really creative work or when I need extra coverage. I'll also use it to completely change a model's skin tone. It's a thick formulation, so I apply by stippling with an Illamasqua Blusher Brush or a damp Beauty Blender.

MAKE UP FOR EVER HD POWDER — This translucent powder is the best. I've been using it constantly since the day I started at makeup school. It never gets cakey, and foundation can easily be applied over it if need be. I use it during shoots to matte any areas where I don't want shine.

CHARLOTTE TILBURY AIRBRUSH FLAWLESS FINISH POWDER — I usually find colored powders too heavy, but I do love this powder by Charlotte Tilbury. I use it when I need a little extra coverage under the eyes or to even out lines on the forehead. It is so fine that it actually blurs away large pores.

MAC PAINT STICKS — MAC Paint Sticks are a big favorite of mine. They can be used for just about anything—lipstick, foundation, blush, eye base.... I use them constantly for creative color work because they blend so seamlessly into foundation and other colors.

ILLAMASQUA GLEAM ——— I mix this into foundation to create amazing glowing skin. I find this cream
IN AURORA makes foundation a shade lighter, so I choose a foundation one shade
darker than the model's natural skin tone.

KEVYN AUCOIN THE ——— Finding a black eye shadow should be simple, but it isn't. Many are bluish
ESSENTIAL EYE SHADOW or have gray tones, and most don't have enough pigment to achieve full
N°110 BLACKEST BLACK coverage. This black eye shadow by Kevyn Aucoin is the real thing; it is
the blackest of black.

MAC EYE KOHL ——— I have been using this wonderful eyeliner by MAC for years. It's so soft
IN SMOLDER that it just glides onto the waterline. And it's a true black—not gray, not
blue. It's perfect.

EYLURE GIRLS ALOUD ——— I usually use individual lashes over strip lashes, but I do love these false lashes
CHERYL FALSE LASHES from Eylure. The strip is almost translucent so you can't see it on camera.

MAC Lip Pencil in Redd
+
Lancôme L'Absolu Rouge 132 Caprice
+
MAC Clear Lipglass
Layer up these three products and you have the reddest, most jaw-dropping
pout on the planet.

Chanel Hydra Beauty Nutrition Baume Nourrissant Lèvres
+
Charlotte Tilbury Light Wonder Foundation
I love a nude lip, but apply foundation directly onto the lips and it is very
drying. To keep lips moist, I mix a small amount of Charlotte Tilbury Light
Wonder Foundation with this beautiful lip balm by Chanel. It creates the
most perfect nude lipstick.

VERA MONA COLOR ——— This clever brush cleaner is my newest obsession. It's a high-tech sponge
SWITCH SOLO that removes eye shadow from brushes with just one or two strokes.
No more running out of clean brushes during a shoot.

Toni's Must-Have Brushes

A QUALITY BRUSH COLLECTION IS VITAL TO A MAKEUP ARTIST'S ARSENAL. THE SMALLER THE BRUSH, THE BETTER, SAYS TONI.

A WELL-THOUGHT-OUT COLLECTION OF BRUSHES IS ESSENTIAL FOR GOOD RESULTS. MY COLLECTION HAS TAKEN ME YEARS OF TRIAL AND ERROR TO BUILD. IT INCLUDES BOTH EXPENSIVE AND BUDGET BRANDS (SUCH AS MY DIY CRAFT BRUSHES), BUT EACH HAS ITS SPECIFIC USE. I USE THEM EVERY DAY AND REALLY COULDN'T WORK WITHOUT THEM.

I'VE LISTED MY FAVORITES. I AM A CONTROL FREAK, SO MY BRUSHES TEND TO BE SMALLER THAN THE ONES MANY OTHER MAKEUP ARTISTS USE. I FIND A SMALLER SIZE ALLOWS ME TO CONTROL EXACTLY WHERE THE PRODUCT GOES.

TIP: BAD BRUSHES JUST MAKE LIFE UNNECESSARILY DIFFICULT. WHEN CHOOSING A BRUSH, GENTLY PUSH THE BRUSH TIP DOWN ON THE BACK OF YOUR HAND. IF THE BRISTLES SPREAD OUT IN ALL DIFFERENT DIRECTIONS, IT MEANS THE BRUSH ISN'T FIRM ENOUGH, WHICH WON'T GIVE YOU THE CONTROL YOU NEED.

FOR COMPLEXION

ILLAMASQUA BLUSHER BRUSH
I like to apply foundation by stippling product into the skin. This brush is perfect for this technique because it not only emulates real pores, it also gives the skin a wonderful skin-plumping lymphatic massage.

MAC 287 DUO FIBRE EYE SHADOW BRUSH
I use this small feathered brush to stipple on foundation or concealer close to the eyes, around the nose, and near the mouth. It blends the product easily and seamlessly into the skin.

SEPHORA 237 BLENDING BRUSH
I am not a fan of using powder unless the look demands it. I mainly use this brush to apply powder around the nose, on and around the eyes, and on the tip of the nose and chin. I like it because it's firm and allows me to remove unwanted shine using very little product. When I do need to mattify the entire face, I still use this brush. It's small but great for pressing powder into the skin.

For Cheeks

Charlotte Tilbury Blusher Brush
Chanel Pinceau Blush Nº 4 Blush Brush

I like to slowly build color by dabbing blush into the cheek, and both these brushes give a seamless application.

Rae Morris Brush 3: Ultimate Cheekbone Brush

I use this brush to apply highlighter above the cheekbone. It applies product in a really beautiful, natural-looking way.

Make Up For Ever Powder Fan Brush 134
Chanel Pinceau Poudre Biseauté Nº 2 Angled Powder Brush

These two brushes have the perfect angle and blend beautifully. I use them to create contour underneath the cheeks.

Sephora Pro Flawless Airbrush #56
MAC 188 Small Duo Fibre Face Brush

I work with MAC Paint Sticks all the time and I find they're best applied with either the Illamasqua Blusher Brush or these two brushes. These fantastic brushes let me stipple and blend the product to achieve a very believable skin-like texture.

For Eyes

Charlotte Tilbury Eye Blender Brush
Make Up For Ever Blender Brush 242

These two brushes make blending eye shadow onto the eyelid so easy. They allow me to slowly build color and blend at the same time.

Rae Morris Brush 7.5: Deluxe Round Shader

This is such a great brush to blend out color over a wide area. I use this to create romantic looks requiring soft color gradations.

Toni's Must-Have Brushes

(continued)

 FOR EYES –

CHARLOTTE TILBURY EYE SMUDGER BRUSH
CHANEL GRAND PINCEAU PAUPIÈRES ROND Nº 19 LARGE BLENDING BRUSH
MAKE UP FOR EVER 216 MEDIUM PRECISION EYE BLENDER BRUSH

These three brushes all blend color beautifully, and they're the perfect size for creating a smoky effect under the lower lashes. I also use them to create extra definition and depth in the creases.

SEPHORA CONCEALER ANTI-CERNE 100 BRUSH

This brush is perfect for applying Chanel's beautiful Illusion D'Ombre eye shadow colors. I use it all the time.

MAC 239 EYE SHADER BRUSH
ILLAMASQUA EYE SHADOW BRUSH

Both of these brushes are able to pack on product to create wonderful dense color.

CHANEL PINCEAU CONTOUR PAUPIÈRES Nº 14 CONTOUR SHADOW BRUSH

I use this brush to add extra definition around the top and bottom lash lines. This brush has changed the way I apply eye makeup—it has made my work so much better.

MAC 228 MINI SHADER BRUSH

I use this brush to apply highlights to the inner corners of the eyes. It is bigger than I would like it to be, but the larger size actually helps me lose a little control over where the product goes, which, in this case, I'm happy about! It gives the application a very organic, unstructured finish.

— Make Up For Ever Extra Fine Eyeliner Brush 250
This eyeliner brush has just the right stiffness to achieve the perfect cat eye.

— MAC 205 Mascara Fan Brush
I love this mascara fan brush. It not only elongates the lashes, it's also fantastic for applying mascara densely at the base of the lashes. It's very precise, too, which allows me to coat mascara onto each individual bottom lash.

— MAC Oval 3 Brush
Some models have small creases under the eyes, and the MAC Oval 3 Brush is perfect for evening out any product that collects in these creases while shooting. A simple swipe over the creases with this brush and any lingering product is gone.

For Lips

— Charlotte Tilbury Lip Brush
Precision is key when creating beautiful lips. This square-ended lip brush makes drawing a perfect lip easy because it gets right into the inner corners of the mouth. I find it so much easier to use than rounded lip brushes.

Credits

SPELLBOUND
Jacket by Amato Haute Couture; headpiece stylist's own.
Photographer: Sylvio Kuehn; **Fashion Stylist:** Lisa Strannesten;
Makeup: Toni Malt.

WILD THING
Blouse by Isabel Marant; jacket by Zara; vintage carpet used
as wrap. **Photographer:** Sylvio Kuehn; **Fashion Stylist:**
Lisa Strannesten; **Makeup & Hair:** Toni Malt; **Makeup & Hair
Assistant:** Katharina Sherman.

HIGH DRAMA
Dress by Michael Cinco Haute Couture; hat by Saint Laurent.
Photographer: Sylvio Kuehn; **Fashion Stylist:** Lisa Strannesten;
Makeup & Hair: Toni Malt; **Makeup & Hair Assistant:**
Katharina Sherman.

ULTRA VIOLET
Jacket by Michael Cinco Couture. **Photographer:** Sylvio Kuehn;
Fashion Stylist: Lisa Strannesten; **Makeup:** Toni Malt.

STARLIGHT
Photographer: Sylvio Kuehn; **Makeup & Hair:** Toni Malt;
Makeup & Hair Assistant: Katharina Sherman.

REBEL INK
Leather jacket by Zara; high-waisted briefs by Dolce & Gabbana.
Photographer: Sylvio Kuehn; **Fashion Stylist:** Lisa Strannesten;
Makeup & Hair: Toni Malt; **Makeup & Hair Assistant:**
Katharina Sherman.

ICE QUEEN
Dress and headpiece by Amato Haute Couture. **Photographer:**
Sylvio Kuehn; **Fashion Stylist:** Lisa Strannesten; **Makeup & Hair:**
Toni Malt; **Makeup & Hair Assistant:** Katharina Sherman.

FELINE SLEEK
Top by Marc Jacobs; hat by Deena & Ozzy. **Photographer:**
Sylvio Kuehn; **Fashion Stylist:** Lisa Strannesten; **Makeup & Hair:**
Toni Malt.

ROCKABILLY GLAMOUR
Photographer: Sylvio Kuehn; **Fashion Stylist:** Lisa Strannesten;
Makeup & Hair: Toni Malt; **Makeup & Hair Assistant:**
Katharina Sherman.

COLOR POP
Dress by Lanvin; loose collar by The Shirt Factory. **Photographer:**
Sylvio Kuehn; **Fashion Stylist:** Lisa Strannesten; **Makeup & Hair:**
Toni Malt; **Makeup & Hair Assistant:** Katharina Sherman.

FADE TO WHITE
Dress by Aiisha Ramadan; coat by Amato Haute Couture; white
dress by Ezra; red dress by Golkar Couture. **Publication:** *Bespoke*;
Photographer: Tina Patni; **Fashion Stylist:** Stuart Robertson;
Makeup & Hair: Toni Malt.

BARE MINIMUM
Blazer by 3.1 Phillip Lim; head wrap made by stylist.
Photographer: Sylvio Kuehn; **Fashion Stylist:** Lisa Strannesten;
Makeup: Toni Malt.

PRECIOUS METAL
Photographer: Sylvio Kuehn; **Makeup:** Toni Malt.

BROWLICIOUS
Top by Theory. **Publication:** *Marie Claire* Arabia; **Photographer:**
Adam Browning-Hill; **Fashion Stylist:** Farah Kabir; **Makeup, Hair
& Nails:** Toni Malt; **Makeup & Hair Assistant:** Katharina Sherman.

COLOR PLAY
Top by Theory. **Publication:** *Marie Claire* Arabia; **Photographer:**
Adam Browning-Hill; **Fashion Stylist:** Farah Kabir; **Makeup & Hair:**
Toni Malt; **Makeup & Hair Assistant:** Katharina Sherman.

SO GLOSSY
Top by Theory. **Publication:** *Marie Claire* Arabia; **Photographer:**
Adam Browning-Hill; **Fashion Stylist:** Farah Kabir; **Makeup & Hair:**
Toni Malt; **Makeup & Hair Assistant:** Katharina Sherman.

HEAT WAVE
Publication: *Marie Claire* Arabia; **Photographer:**
Adam Browning-Hill; **Fashion Stylist:** Farah Kabir; **Makeup & Hair:**
Toni Malt; **Makeup & Hair Assistant:** Katharina Sherman.

THE BIG BLEND
Top by Issa. **Publication:** *Marie Claire* Arabia; **Photographer:**
Adam Browning-Hill; **Fashion Stylist:** Farah Kabir; **Makeup & Hair:**
Toni Malt; **Makeup & Hair Assistant:** Katharina Sherman.

IN FULL BLOOM
Blouse by Joie; headpiece stylist's own; vintage hood.
Photographer: Sylvio Kuehn; **Fashion Stylist:** Lisa Strannesten;
Makeup & Hair: Toni Malt.

POWER PLAY
Blazer by Alice + Olivia. **Photographer:** Sylvio Kuehn; **Fashion
Stylist:** Lisa Strannesten; **Makeup & Hair:** Toni Malt; **Makeup & Hair
Assistant:** Katharina Sherman.

FLOAT AWAY WITH ME
Bathing suit by Melissa Odabash. **Photographer:** Sylvio Kuehn; **Fashion Stylist:** Lisa Strannesten; **Makeup & Hair:** Toni Malt.

SHADOW PLAY
Photographer: Sylvio Kuehn; **Makeup:** Toni Malt.

SPARKLE AND SHINE
Mickey Mouse–embellished college sweater by Marc Jacobs; high-waisted briefs by Sonia Rykiel; shoes by Charlotte Olympia. **Photographer:** Sylvio Kuehn; **Fashion Stylist:** Lisa Strannesten; **Makeup & Hair:** Toni Malt; **Makeup & Hair Assistant:** Katharina Sherman.

WILD ONE
Sequin jacket by Gryphon; shirt by Diane von Furstenberg; shorts by Topshop; bracelets by Eddie Borgo & J. Dauphin. **Photographer:** Sylvio Kuehn; **Fashion Stylist:** Lisa Strannesten; **Makeup & Hair:** Toni Malt.

ON THE EDGE
Photographer: Sylvio Kuehn; **Makeup & Hair:** Toni Malt.

BOMBSHELL RED
High-waisted briefs and bra by Dolce & Gabbana; stockings by Falke; shoes by Charlotte Olympia. **Photographer:** Sylvio Kuehn; **Fashion Stylist:** Lisa Strannesten; **Makeup:** Toni Malt; **Hair:** Katharina Sherman.

CALIFORNIA DREAMING
Tank top by Isabel Marant; bra by H&M; chinos by Rag & Bone; vintage belt by Dolce & Gabbana; shoes by Converse; earrings by Kenneth Jay Lane. **Photographer:** Sylvio Kuehn; **Fashion Stylist:** Lisa Strannesten; **Makeup & Hair:** Toni Malt; **Makeup & Hair Assistant:** Katharina Sherman.

DREAM WEAVER
Dress by Amato Haute Couture. **Photographer:** Sylvio Kuehn; **Fashion Stylist:** Lisa Strannesten; **Makeup & Hair:** Toni Malt; **Hair Assistant:** Katharina Sherman.

JAPANESE LOVE STORY
Vest by Zara; shorts by Sonia Rykiel; obi belt stylist's own. **Photographer:** Sylvio Kuehn; **Fashion Stylist:** Lisa Strannesten; **Makeup & Hair:** Toni Malt; **Makeup & Hair Assistant:** Katharina Sherman.

FUTURE SHOCK
Jacket by Amato Haute Couture. **Photographer:** Sylvio Kuehn; **Fashion Stylist:** Lisa Strannesten; **Makeup & Hair:** Toni Malt; **Makeup & Hair Assistant:** Katharina Sherman.

GLAMAZON GOLD
Dress by Ezra. **Photographer:** Sylvio Kuehn; **Fashion Stylist:** Lisa Strannesten; **Makeup & Hair:** Toni Malt; **Makeup & Hair Assistant:** Katharina Sherman.

LACE UP
Photographer: Sylvio Kuehn; **Makeup:** Toni Malt.

FIRST FLUSH
Photographer: Sylvio Kuehn; **Makeup:** Toni Malt.

GOLD RUSH
Dress by Amato Haute Couture. **Photographer:** Sylvio Kuehn; **Fashion Stylist:** Lisa Strannesten; **Makeup & Hair:** Toni Malt.

WET, WET, WET
Outfit by Nike. **Photographer:** Sylvio Kuehn; **Fashion Stylist:** Lisa Strannesten; **Makeup & Hair:** Toni Malt.

COLOR RUSH
Photographer: Sylvio Kuehn; **Fashion Stylist:** Lisa Strannesten; **Makeup & Hair:** Toni Malt.

LIGHT FANTASTIC
Photographer: Sylvio Kuehn; **Fashion Stylist:** Lisa Strannesten; **Makeup:** Toni Malt.

SCARLET FEVER
Dress by Amato Haute Couture. **Photographer:** Sylvio Kuehn; **Fashion Stylist:** Lisa Strannesten; **Makeup & Hair:** Toni Malt; **Makeup & Hair Assistant:** Katharina Sherman.

SHADES OF GRAY
Dress by Jason Wu; earrings by Michael Cinco Haute Couture. **Photographer:** Sylvio Kuehn; **Fashion Stylist:** Lisa Strannesten; **Makeup & Hair:** Toni Malt.

POP TO IT
Yellow jacket by Marc Jacobs; striped pants by True Religion; blazer and shorts by Paul & Joe; yellow set with sequins by Marc Jacobs. **Photographer:** Sylvio Kuehn; **Fashion Stylist:** Lisa Strannesten; **Makeup & Hair:** Toni Malt; **Makeup & Hair Assistant:** Katharina Sherman.

Credits

(continued)

LOUD MOUTH
Photographer: Sylvio Kuehn; **Makeup:** Toni Malt.

BOOGIE NIGHTS
Photographer: Sylvio Kuehn; **Fashion Stylist:** Lisa Strannesten;
Makeup & Hair: Toni Malt; **Makeup & Hair Assistant:**
Katharina Sherman.

THE NEW MATTE
Dress by Amato Haute Couture. **Photographer:** Sylvio Kuehn;
Fashion Stylist: Lisa Strannesten; **Makeup & Hair:** Toni Malt;
Hair Assistant: Katharina Sherman.

SIMPLY RED (ALSO FEATURED ON PAGES 6–7)
Photographer: Sylvio Kuehn; **Makeup:** Toni Malt.

A WINTER'S TALE
Dress and jacket by Diane von Furstenberg; fur collar by Paule Ka.
Photographer: Sylvio Kuehn; **Fashion Stylist:** Lisa Strannesten;
Makeup: Toni Malt; **Hair:** Katharina Sherman.

ABOUT A BOY
Shirt by Reitmayer; vintage bow tie by Bambah Boutique;
jacket by Zara. **Photographer:** Sylvio Kuehn; **Fashion Stylist:**
Lisa Strannesten; **Makeup:** Toni Malt; **Hair:** Katharina Sherman.

COLOR BLAST
Photographer: Sylvio Kuehn; **Fashion Stylist:** Lisa Strannesten;
Makeup & Hair: Toni Malt; **Makeup & Hair Assistant:**
Katharina Sherman.

SURREALIST BLUE
Blouse and scarf by Isabel Marant; vintage necklace and skirt
made by stylist. **Photographer:** Sylvio Kuehn; **Fashion Stylist:**
Lisa Strannesten; **Makeup & Hair:** Toni Malt; **Makeup & Hair
Assistant:** Katharina Sherman.

FAIRY DUST
Photographer: Sylvio Kuehn; **Makeup:** Toni Malt.

DARK ROMANCE
Embellished hood and cape by Michael Cinco Haute Couture.
Photographer: Sylvio Kuehn; **Fashion Stylist:** Lisa Strannesten;
Makeup & Hair: Toni Malt.

BLINK!
Dress by Marc Jacobs. **Photographer:** Sylvio Kuehn;
Fashion Stylist: Lisa Strannesten; **Makeup & Hair:** Toni Malt.

BLACK MAGIC
Dress by Michael Cinco. **Photographer:** Sylvio Kuehn;
Fashion Stylist: Lisa Strannesten; **Makeup:** Toni Malt;
Makeup & Hair Assistant: Katharina Sherman.

WITH THE BAND
Print coat by Alaïa; cropped turtleneck top by Topshop; pencil
skirt and belt by Ralph Lauren; earrings by Anne Gedeon; bracelet
by Michael Kors; rings by Miriam Salat. **Publication:** *Rolling Stone*;
Photographer: Tina Chang; **Fashion Stylist:** Claire Carruthers;
Makeup & Hair: Toni Malt.

PRECIOUS GEMS
Photographer: Sylvio Kuehn; **Makeup:** Toni Malt.

HEAVY METAL
Blazer and trousers by Theyskens' Theory; vintage boa and nose
ring stylist's own. **Photographer:** Sylvio Kuehn; **Fashion Stylist:**
Lisa Strannesten; **Makeup:** Toni Malt; **Hair:** Katharina Sherman.

INTO THE BLUE
Photographer: Sylvio Kuehn; **Makeup:** Toni Malt.

BELLE DU JOUR
Top by Marc Jacobs; hat by Deena & Ozzy.
Photographer: Sylvio Kuehn; **Fashion Stylist:** Lisa Strannesten;
Makeup & Hair: Toni Malt.

INTO THE LIGHT
All clothes and makeup by Chanel. **Publication:** *Sayidaty*;
Photographer: Mazen Abusrour; **Fashion Stylist:** Claire Carruthers;
Makeup: Toni Malt; **Hair:** Lorna Butler.

RAY OF LIGHT
Necklace by Michael Cinco Haute Couture; headpiece
stylist's own. **Photographer:** Sylvio Kuehn;
Fashion Stylist: Lisa Strannesten; **Makeup:** Toni Malt.

BODY BEAUTIFUL
Outfit by Nike. **Photographer:** Adam Browning-Hill;
Fashion Stylist: Lisa Strannesten; **Makeup & Hair:** Toni Malt.

PAGE 9, MEET SOPHIA

Publication: *Sayidaty*; **Photographer:** Mazen Abusrour;
Fashion Stylist: Claire Carruthers; **Makeup:** Toni Malt;
Hair: Lorna Butler.

PAGE 10, ABOUT TONI

Photographer: Sylvio Kuehn.

PAGE 12, LOOKS

All clothes and makeup by Chanel. **Publication:** *Sayidaty*;
Photographer: Mazen Abusrour; **Fashion Stylist:** Claire Carruthers;
Makeup: Toni Malt; **Hair:** Lorna Butler.

PAGES 156-57, MAGAZINE COVERS

Top row, from left to right:

1) **Publication:** *Vogue* India; **Photographer:** Mazen Abusrour;
Fashion Stylist: Anaita Adajania; **Makeup & Hair:** Toni Malt;
Model: Eva Doll.

2) **Publication:** *Glamour* Iceland; **Photographer:** Silja Magg;
Fashion Stylist: Ina Lekiewicz; **Makeup:** Toni Malt;
Hair: Pablo Kuemin; **Model:** Coco Rocha.

3) **Publication:** *Harper's Bazaar* Arabia; **Photographer:** Silja Magg;
Fashion Stylist: Katie Trotter; **Makeup & Hair:** Toni Malt;
Model: Chanel Iman.

4) **Publication:** *Elle* Middle East; **Photographer:** Greg Adamski;
Fashion Stylist: Ghina Maalouf; **Makeup:** Toni Malt;
Hair: Melanie Meyer; **Model:** Anna Yve.

5) **Publication:** *Harper's Bazaar* Arabia;
Photographer: Silja Magg; **Fashion Stylist:** Katie Trotter;
Makeup: Toni Malt; **Hair:** Adrian Clark; **Model:** Nina Abdel Malak.

6) **Publication:** *Harper's Bazaar* Arabia;
Photographer: Silja Magg; **Fashion Stylist:** Katie Trotter;
Makeup: Toni Malt, **Hair:** Adrian Clark; **Model:** Nina Abdel Malak.

Middle row, from left to right:

1) **Publication:** *Marie Claire* Lower Gulf;
Photographer: Pelle Lannefors; **Fashion Stylist:** Sarah Rasheed;
Makeup & Hair: Toni Malt; **Model:** Beata Grabowska.

2) **Publication:** *Harper's Bazaar* Arabia;
Photographer: Mathieu Cesar; **Fashion Stylist:** Sally Matthews;
Makeup: Toni Malt; **Hair:** Frederic Barat; **Model:** Freida Pinto.

3) **Publication:** *Harper's Bazaar* Arabia;
Photographer: Adam Browning-Hill;
Fashion Stylist: Katie Trotter; **Makeup:** Toni Malt;
Hair: Annesofie Begtrup; **Model:** Samira Mahboub.

4) **Publication:** *Vogue* India; **Photographer:** Tejal Patni;
Fashion Stylist: Anaita Adajania; **Makeup:** Toni Malt;
Hair: Manuel Losada; **Model:** Shraddha Kapoor.

5) **Publication:** *Glamour* Iceland; **Photographer:** Silja Magg;
Fashion Stylist: Ina Lekiewicz; **Makeup:** Toni Malt;
Hair: Pablo Kuemin; **Model:** Coco Rocha.
6) **Publication:** *Harper's Bazaar* Arabia;
Photographer: Rene & Radka; **Fashion Stylist:** Katie Trotter;
Makeup: Toni Malt; **Hair:** Pablo Kuemin; **Model:** Jessica Kahawaty.

Bottom row, from left to right:

1) **Publication:** *Harper's Bazaar* Arabia; **Photographer:** Silja Magg;
Fashion Stylist: Katie Trotter; **Makeup & Hair:** Toni Malt;
Model: Chanel Iman.

2) **Publication:** *Harper's Bazaar* Arabia; **Photographer:** Silja Magg;
Fashion Stylist: Katie Trotter; **Makeup:** Toni Malt; **Hair:** Seiji;
Models: Jourdana Phillips, Grace Mahary, Ajak Deng, Lameka Fox,
Nykhor-Nyakueinyang Paul.

3) **Publication:** *Luxury*; **Photographer:** Greg Adamski;
Fashion Stylist: Katie Trotter; **Makeup & Hair:** Toni Malt;
Model: Angelika Maciolek.

4) **Publication:** *Marie Claire* Lower Gulf;
Photographer: Pelle Lannefors; **Fashion Stylist:** Sarah Rasheed;
Makeup & Hair: Toni Malt; **Model:** Ilona Novacek.

5) **Publication:** *Harper's Bazaar* Arabia;
Photographer: Silja Magg; **Fashion Stylist:** Katie Trotter;
Makeup & Hair: Toni Malt; **Model:** Dorota Kullova.

6) **Publication:** *Harper's Bazaar* Arabia;
Photographer: Adam Browning-Hill; **Fashion Stylist:** Katie Trotter;
Makeup: Toni Malt; **Hair:** Annesofie Degtrup;
Model: Samira Mahboub.

PAGE 160, INSIDE TONI'S KIT

Photographer: Adam Browning-Hill.

Acknowledgments

My sincere thanks and gratitude go out to Esther Kremer, Lindsey Tulloch, and the team of Assouline for their support and guidance throughout the crucial final stage of *Transform*. You all made my dream reality.

I would also like to thank my extraordinarily supportive and truly brilliant retoucher, Victor Wagner, whose skill always far surpasses expectations. I am still convinced that he was a makeup artist in his previous life.

My sincere appreciation is extended to my incredibly gifted copy editor Sally Hunwick, who always found the most beautiful words. You transformed my thoughts into wonderful stories that I continue to love reading.

Thank you to Maliha Al Tabari, whose passion and motivation are so infectious. You gave me the courage to think big.

Special thanks to Soha Nashaat for always encouraging me and always moving mountains to help.

Assouline would like to thank Phyllis Fong and Zach Townsend for their contributions to this book.

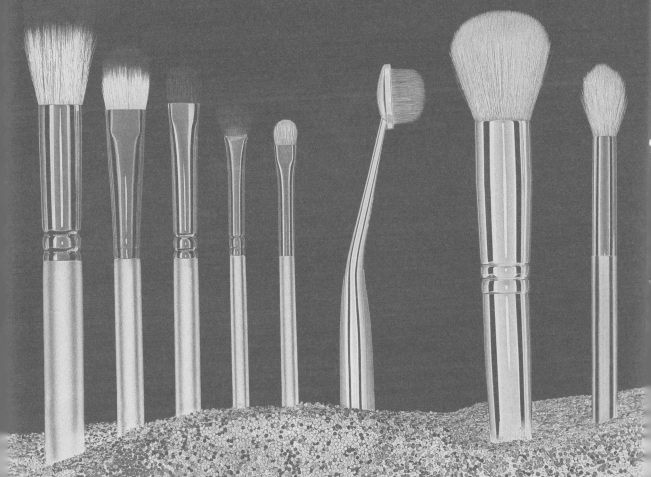